DIABETES & PREGNANCY

A Guide to a Healthy Pregnancy
for Women Who Have
Type 1, Type 2, or Gestational Diabetes

DAVID A. SACKS, MD
EDITOR

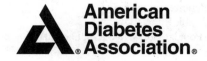

American Diabetes Association®

Director, Book Publishing, Abe Ogden; Managing Editor, Greg Guthrie; Acquisitions Editor, Victor Van Beuren; Editor, Rebekah Renshaw; Production Manager, Melissa Sprott; Composition, ADA; Cover Design, pixiedesign, llc.; Printer, Victor Graphics.

Printed in the United States of America
1 3 5 7 9 10 8 6 4 2

The suggestions and information contained in this publication are generally consistent with the *Clinical Practice Recommendations* and other policies of the American Diabetes Association, but they do not represent the policy or position of the Association or any of its boards or committees. Reasonable steps have been taken to ensure the accuracy of the information presented. However, the American Diabetes Association cannot ensure the safety or efficacy of any product or service described in this publication. Individuals are advised to consult a physician or other appropriate health care professional before undertaking any diet or exercise program or taking any medication referred to in this publication. Professionals must use and apply their own professional judgment, experience, and training and should not rely solely on the information contained in this publication before prescribing any diet, exercise, or medication. The American Diabetes Association— its officers, directors, employees, volunteers, and members—assumes no responsibility or liability for personal or other injury, loss, or damage that may result from the suggestions or information in this publication.

⊚ The paper in this publication meets the requirements of the ANSI Standard Z39.48-1992 (permanence of paper).

ADA titles may be purchased for business or promotional use or for special sales. To purchase more than 50 copies of this book at a discount, or for custom editions of this book with your logo, contact the American Diabetes Association at the address below, at booksales@diabetes. org, or by calling 703-299-2046.

American Diabetes Association
1701 North Beauregard Street
Alexandria, Virginia 22311

DOI: 10.2337/9781580404372

Library of Congress Cataloging-in-Publication Data

Diabetes and pregnancy : a guide to a healthy pregnancy for women with type 1, type 2, or gestational diabetes / [edited by] David A. Sacks.
    p. cm.
Includes bibliographical references and index.
ISBN 978-1-58040-437-2 (pbk.)
1. Diabetes in pregnancy--Popular works. I. Sacks, David A.
RG580.D5D513 2011
618.3'64--dc22

2011014144

Dedication

This book is dedicated to all reproductive age women who have some form of diabetes, and to those who may develop diabetes. We hope that its contents will provide you with knowledge that will enable you to help you have the best outcome possible before, during, and after your pregnancy.

Table of Contents

Acknowledgments

This book is intended as an update and combining of two previous publications (*Diabetes & Pregnancy: What to Expect, 4th ed.* and *Gestational Diabetes: What to Expect, 5th ed.*). The reason for combining these books was that gestational diabetes in many instances will develop into permanent diabetes. This is important to know because it is now possible to decrease your risks of developing diabetes in the years following pregnancy. We are grateful to the authors, editors, and reviewers of the many editions of both these texts for having provided the template for the current book.

The editor wishes to personally express his gratitude to all the contributors to this book. Largely academic clinicians, they bravely undertook the task of taking some fairly sophisticated medical concepts and translating them into everyday language.

Recognition is also extended to the "behind the scenes" people without whom this publication would remain a sequence of ideas united by a sequence of bits and bytes on a computer. Special thanks go to Rebekah Renshaw, developmental editor; Victor Van Beuren, acquisitions; and Abe Ogden, director of book publishing, of the ADA for their support and counsel throughout the development of this book.

Thanks also to the reviewers of this book: Boyd Metzger, MD; Martha Funnell, MS, RN, CDE; Florence Brown, MD; Sue Kirkman, MD; and Stephanie Dunbar, RD.

—*David A. Sacks, MD*

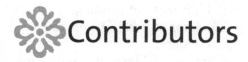Contributors

Howard Berger, MD
Head, Maternal Fetal Medicine
St. Michael's Hospital
Assistant Professor
University of Toronto
Toronto, Canada

Kathleen M. Berkowitz, MD
Medical Director, Maternal
Transport Program
MemorialCare Center for
Women at Miller Children's
Hospital & Long Beach
Memorial Medical Center

Denice Feig, MD, MSc
Associate Professor
Departments of Medicine,
Obstetrics & Gynecology,
Health Policy, Management &
Evaluation
University of Toronto,
Mount Sinai Hospital
Toronto, Canada

T. Murphy Goodwin, MD
Professor of Obstetrics and
Gynecology and Pediatrics
Chief, Maternal-Fetal Medicine
University of
Southern California

Mandhir Gupta, MD
Director NICU and
Assistant Chief Pediatrics
Kaiser Permanente

Susan Hales, RD, CDE
Perinatal Diabetes Center
Cabell Huntington Hospital
Huntington, West Virginia

Janet C. King, PhD
Senior Scientist
Children's Hospital Oakland
Research Institute
Oakland, California
Professor
University of California
Berkeley & Davis

Martin Montoro, MD
Professor of Clinical Medicine
& OB/GYN
Division of Maternal-Fetal
Medicine
Keck School of Medicine
University of
Southern California

Laura Mullarky, RN, CDE
Perinatal Diabetes Center
Cabell Huntington Hospital
Huntington, West Virginia

Robin Reeves, BSN
Coordinator Perinatal Center
Cabell Huntington Hospital
Huntington, West Virginia

Carolina Reyes, MD
Clinical Associate Professor
Maternal-Fetal Medicine
Keck School of Medicine
University of Southern
California
Maternal-Fetal Medicine
Virginia Hospital Center
Arlington, Virginia

Barak M. Rosenn, MD
Professor of Clinical Obstetrics
and Gynecology
Columbia University College
of Physicians and Surgeons
Director of Obstetrics and
Maternal-Fetal Medicine
St. Luke's Roosevelt
Hospital Center
New York, New York

Penina Segall-Gutierrez, MD, MSc
Assistant Professor of Clinical
Obstetrics and Gynecology
and Family Medicine
Keck School of Medicine
University of
Southern California

Shailini Singh, MD
Clinical Professor of OB/GYN
University of Buffalo
Director of Fetal Diagnostic
Center
Director of Metabolic Syndrome
Center
Kaleida Health Care
Former Director of
Perinatal Center and Perinatal
Diabetes Center
Cabell Huntington Hospital
Huntington, West Virginia

Naomi E. Stotland, MD
Associate Professor
Department of Obstetrics,
Gynecology, and Reproductive
Sciences
University of California,
San Francisco

Bonnie Trader, RN
Perinatal Diabetes Center
Cabell Huntington Hospital
Huntington, West Virginia

Terri Weiland, RN, CDE
Diabetes and Pregnancy
Case Manager
WCH High Risk Services

Introduction

This book is for any woman who has diabetes and who is, or will soon be, of an age when she is capable of having babies. It started as a project to combine and update two earlier books published by the American Diabetes Association, one of which deals with pregnancy for women who had diabetes before they got pregnant, and the other for women whose diabetes first occurred or was first recognized during pregnancy. It subsequently took on a personal aspect, because as the chapters came in, I found myself wishing that my patients had access to this information before they became pregnant.

The time to begin care for pregnancy for a woman who has diabetes or who is at high risk for developing diabetes while pregnant is *before* she becomes pregnant. The book contains information about why having diabetes requires special preparation for pregnancy, how important it is to use a reliable family planning method until pregnancy is desired, and how to get yourself and your blood glucose levels into the best shape possible before getting pregnant. It also covers what the medical professionals working with you will do for and with you while preparing for and during your pregnancy.

The authors and contributors to this book come from different parts of the medical world: perinatologists, neonatologists, generalists, endocrinologists, and diabetes nurse-educators. They (and I) have two things in common: We are all members of the diabetes in pregnancy teams at our respective medical centers, and we all believe that by your being informed about what should be done to protect your health before and during your pregnancy, you will greatly increase the probability of your having a healthy baby and a healthy you.

Hopefully this book will help you understand all that's involved in preparing for and caring for yourself during your pregnancy. There will be changes you'll be asked to make. Perhaps you will find yourself eating new foods and cutting out some foods that you really like. Daily exercise may be a new addition to your life. Taking a few minutes four or more times a day to check your blood glucose may require educating your family, friends, and employer about the need for time to perform this task. Diabetes doesn't give you any days off—you have to follow the program every day. You are the head of your health care team and your pregnancy. Your health care providers are here to help you and your baby to be as healthy as possible.

David A. Sacks, MD
Adjunct Investigator
Department of Research and Evaluation
Kaiser Permanente Southern California
Pasadena, California
Clinical Professor
Department of Obstetrics and Gynecology
University of Southern California
Keck School of Medicine
Los Angeles, California

Chapter 1

How Can Diabetes Affect My Baby and Me?

Pregnancy is a time of change and excitement. So many things in your life will change and taking care of yourself and your baby will be the most important part of your life. The last thing you want to think about is diabetes and how it will affect you and your baby! The great news is that women who manage their diabetes well during pregnancy can have a relatively normal pregnancy and give birth to a healthy baby.

Working with a health care team is an important part of staying healthy during your pregnancy. The members of this team usually include a doctor, a nurse, a diabetes educator, a dietitian, and a social worker. Each of them is concerned with different aspects of your care, and each will be available to you as your pregnancy, or preparation for pregnancy, advances. The captain of the team is....YOU! Everything your team members do is for *your* health and the health of *your* baby.

Before we talk about planning for pregnancy, it's good to first understand diabetes. If you had diabetes before your pregnancy, you may already be familiar with what diabetes is and the different types of diabetes. If you are pregnant and recently diagnosed with gestational diabetes, you may have no idea what the diagnosis means for you, your baby, and your future. This chapter will focus on the different types of diabetes, risk factors for developing diabetes, and how having diabetes will have an effect on your pregnancy. It's important to remember that with careful management, you and your baby can both have a healthy, happy long life.

What Is Diabetes?

Diabetes is a disorder where the body does not produce insulin or doesn't use the insulin it produces properly. Insulin is a hormone made in your pancreas that allows the foods you eat to be turned into energy and energy reserves that your body uses for fuel. Food is eventually converted into glucose (a simple sugar). Your body needs insulin to turn the foods you eat into energy that fuels your body.

People who have diabetes have difficulty naturally regulating their blood glucose levels, either because they don't produce enough insulin or because they are unable to use insulin properly. When your body is unable to properly respond to the insulin that is made, this is known as insulin resistance. When insulin doesn't work correctly, your blood glucose levels will rise. High blood glucose levels can damage blood vessels in different organs, which may result in those organs working less effectively than they should.

Diabetes is increasingly common, likely due to rising rates of obesity in developed and some underdeveloped countries. As of 2011, 25.8 million children and adults in the U.S.—8.3% of the population—have diabetes. Over 18 million people have been diagnosed, while 7 million people don't even know they are living with diabetes and are undiagnosed.

Diabetes Statistics

▶ 25.8 million children and adults in the U.S. have diabetes—8.3% of the population.

▶ Men: 13 million, or 11.8% of all men age 20 years or older, have diabetes.

▶ Women: 12.6 million, or 10.8% of all women age 20 years or older, have diabetes.

▶ 18.8 million Americans have been diagnosed while 7 million Americans remain undiagnosed.

▶ 1.9 million new cases of diabetes were diagnosed in people age 20 or over in 2010.

According to the National Diabetes Fact Sheet, 2011.

Diabetes is dangerous because people affected with the most common form of this disease may not know that they have it. A person may have blood glucose levels that are high and not know it, because he or she feels fine. However, if blood glucose levels are allowed to remain elevated for prolonged periods of time, it may cause serious consequences, such as heart attack, high blood pressure, stroke, blindness, and loss of limbs. While it is potentially a very dangerous condition, with proper management, including lifestyle changes and use of medications, diabetes can be successfully managed and its complications prevented.

Types of Diabetes

The three main types of diabetes are type 1, type 2, and gestational. Type 2 is the most common type of diabetes in non-pregnant people. In the U.S., type 1 is found in about 1% of pregnant women. Type 2 is found in only about 10% of pregnant women who have diabetes. The other 90% have gestational diabetes. Gestational diabetes is a form of diabetes that is diagnosed during pregnancy, and usually goes away after delivery. All three types, their risk factors, and common symptoms are explained further below.

TYPE 2 DIABETES—THE "INSULIN-RESISTANT" DIABETES

Type 2 diabetes is the most common type of diabetes. About 90–95% of people with diabetes have type 2. Type 2 diabetes used to be known as "adult onset diabetes"; however, in recent years, more children and teens have started developing type 2.

Type 2 diabetes typically doesn't have a rapid onset. You may not have noticeable symptoms, or you may only have mild symptoms for years before you are diagnosed with diabetes. Type 2 is often diagnosed during a routine exam or blood test. People with type 2 often still produce insulin, especially when they are first diagnosed.

Most people with type 2 diabetes have insulin resistance (are unable to use the insulin they do produce properly). Over time, the pancreas (the organ in which insulin is made) cannot keep up, blood glucose levels rise, and diabetes develops. It's the fall in insulin production that leads to diabetes. People who are insulin resistant but can produce enough insulin have normal blood glucose levels. This insulin resistance may be inherited; however, it may also be triggered by unhealthy choices, such as lack of physical activity and/or excessive weight gain. After years of producing excess amounts of insulin, the pancreas cannot keep up with the greater requirements. When diabetes is poorly controlled, it's more difficult to conceive, but is still possible.

Common Symptoms of Type 2 Diabetes

When blood glucose levels are only modestly high, you may have no symptoms at all. Very elevated blood glucose levels can cause:

▶ Frequent urination—due to the body trying to flush out excess glucose

▶ Increased thirst—due to dehydration

▶ Fatigue—because glucose is not getting to your cells properly

▶ Blurred vision—due to a buildup of fluid in your eyes or increased glucose levels

▶ Slow healing of infections of the skin

▶ Yeast infections, such as vaginal infections

There are several risk factors that increase the likelihood of developing type 2 diabetes. The most common are a combination of heredity, ethnic origin, excess weight, sedentary lifestyle, history of gestational diabetes, and having given birth to a baby over 9 pounds.

Type 2 diabetes can be managed through healthy eating, physical activity, and blood glucose–lowering medications (pills or insulin). There are a number of treatment options for managing type 2 diabetes. How you manage your diabetes depends on your personal goals. Work with your health care providers to come up with a plan for managing your diabetes and meeting those goals.

TYPE 1 DIABETES—THE "ABSENT INSULIN" DIABETES

Type 1 diabetes is less common than type 2 in the overall population. Type 1 used to be called "juvenile-onset" diabetes because it is most often diagnosed in childhood or early teen years; however, it can be diagnosed well into adulthood.

People with type 1 diabetes produce very little or no insulin because their insulin-producing cells in the pancreas have been destroyed. Because they no longer produce enough insulin, people with type 1 diabetes need to take insulin, in the form of either injections or an insulin pump.

The destruction of these cells is due to cell-destroying processes related to the immune system (called auto-immunity). This autoimmune response makes the body turn on itself and attack the insulin-making cells (β-cells) in the pancreas. It is not known what triggers the autoimmune attack, but genetic factors and "environmental" factors, such as viral infections, play a role.

Because people with type 1 diabetes produce little to no insulin, blood glucose levels often rise swiftly and symptoms are often serious when they appear. Most people when they are diagnosed with type 1 feel very sick and are often rushed to the hospital because their symptoms are so severe.

Symptoms of Type 1 Diabetes

▶ Frequent urination

▶ Increased thirst

▶ Fatigue

▶ Blurred vision

▶ Weight loss (even with increased appetite)

▶ Nausea and vomiting

There is no way to prevent type 1 but scientists and researchers are investigating how to delay or reduce the severity of type 1 diabetes.

Management of type 1 diabetes is typically a combination of insulin, healthy eating, and exercise; however, how you manage your diabetes depends on your personal goals. Insulin is necessary because your body does not produce the needed amount. Exercise lowers your blood glucose level, so physical activity can help reduce the amount of insulin you need to take. Even though type 1 diabetes can be difficult to manage, pregnancy can be successful with careful treatment. Getting your blood glucose levels as close to normal as possible before getting pregnant can go a long way toward making sure you and your baby remain healthy (see chapter 2).

GESTATIONAL DIABETES

Gestational diabetes is a type of diabetes that comes on during pregnancy and usually goes away after delivery. Gestational diabetes is the most common type of diabetes during pregnancy. Gestational diabetes affects about 4% of all pregnant women—about 135,000 cases of gestational diabetes in the United States each year. Gestational diabetes refers only to diabetes in women who have never had diabetes before and develop high blood glucose during pregnancy. It does not refer to women with pre-existing type 1 or type 2 diabetes who become pregnant.

Gestational diabetes usually develops during the second trimester of a pregnancy. This is the time when hormones of pregnancy naturally begin to cause changes in how your body uses insulin. Pregnancy causes many changes in your metabolism, including a state of insulin resistance similar to type 2 diabetes. This insulin resistance usually increases as pregnancy advances.

The insulin resistance of pregnancy helps the mother transfer nutrients from her blood to the blood of the baby. Most women can produce the

Risk Factors for Developing Gestational Diabetes

▶ Mothers 35 years or older

▶ Having a close family member with diabetes

▶ Having had gestational diabetes in a previous pregnancy

▶ Being overweight or obese

▶ Having polycystic ovary disease

▶ Complications in a previous pregnancy such as having had a large baby, a stillborn baby, or a baby born with malformations

▶ Women who are African American, Latina, Pacific Islander, Native American, or Asian

extra insulin needed to compensate for these changes unique to pregnancy. However, women who have diabetes during pregnancy cannot produce the extra insulin needed to maintain a healthy blood glucose level. Because of this, the mother's blood glucose levels remain too high and too much glucose is transferred to the baby. This can cause the baby to become too big, as well as other problems.

It is difficult to detect gestational diabetes without a blood test because there are no outward symptoms. The American Diabetes Association recommends that all pregnant women be screened for gestational diabetes between 24 and 28 weeks of pregnancy with a test called an oral glucose tolerance test (see How Diabetes Is Diagnosed, below).

For most women who have gestational diabetes, blood glucose levels return to normal after giving birth. However, if you have had gestational diabetes, your risk of developing type 2 diabetes at some time in the future when you are no longer pregnant is increased. After having gestational diabetes, your child may also be at increased risk of developing obesity and type 2 diabetes at some time during childhood or (more commonly) adulthood. The good news is that by limiting your weight gain and keeping your blood glucose levels close to normal, you may decrease the risk of these adverse outcomes for both you and your child.

The potential complications of gestational diabetes for both you and your baby are similar to those for pregnant women with type 1 and type 2 diabetes (see chapter 3), except that the risk of birth defects is not increased, since high blood glucose develops in gestational diabetes after the baby's organs are completely formed. Most of the time gestational diabetes may be treated with only a change in diet and an increase in daily exercise (See chapter 5). Sometimes, despite following diet and activity instructions to the letter, you may require insulin injections (see chapter 4) to lower your blood glucose. Discuss your treatment options with your health care team.

How Diabetes Is Diagnosed

You may have already been diagnosed with type 1 or type 2 diabetes before you were pregnant. Although you or your health care provider may suspect you have type 2 diabetes, the only way to know for sure is to have your blood glucose tested. If you are pregnant and have risk factors for type 2 diabetes, your doctor should do a blood test for type 2 diabetes at your first prenatal visit. If you do not have diabetes already, you should be tested for gestational diabetes at 24–28 weeks into your pregnancy.

There are four different tests for diagnosing type 1 or type 2 diabetes: A1C, fasting plasma glucose test, random plasma glucose test, and oral glucose tolerance test. Gestational diabetes may be diagnosed with a glucose tolerance test, or if a fasting glucose level meets certain values (92–125 mg/dl).

In the A1C test, a small sample of blood is collected from a vein. The test measures the concentration of hemoglobin molecules that have glucose attached to them. Hemoglobin is the material in the red blood cells that carries oxygen. The glucose attached to hemoglobin does not affect its ability to do this. The A1C represents a measure of blood glucose levels over the past 2–3 months and is given as a percentage. An A1C greater than 6.5% (repeated to confirm the result) is used to diagnose diabetes. This test can be used to diagnose diabetes prior to pregnancy, or to detect type 2 at your first prenatal visit, but it cannot be used to diagnose gestational diabetes.

The fasting plasma glucose test measures the amount of glucose in the blood after not eating for 8–10 hours. A firm diagnosis is made when two tests (done on different days) are at least 126 mg/dl. The random glucose test also measures the amount of glucose in the blood, but is done at a random time without fasting. You may be diagnosed with diabetes if your blood glucose is at or above 200 mg/dl and you have symptoms of diabetes.

The oral glucose tolerance test is used to test for gestational diabetes, but can be used to test for other types of diabetes as well. This test takes two hours. You should not eat or drink anything except water, from midnight of the night before the test until you complete the test. A sample of blood will be drawn. Next, you will drink a glucose solution that tastes like a sweet soda and have a sample of blood drawn one and two hours after drinking the glucose solution.

The Dangers of Diabetes During Pregnancy

Most women with diabetes who manage their glucose levels have healthy babies; however, if you do not actively care for your diabetes during pregnancy, there are significant risks to you and the baby.

If you had type 1 or type 2 diabetes before getting pregnant, maintaining blood glucose levels and A1C close to normal just before and during the first trimester (the first three months) is critical to the proper development of the child while in the mother's womb. High blood glucose levels during the first trimester—the time when the baby's organs are forming—increase the risk of birth defects and also miscarriage. Since the baby's organs are completely formed by 7 weeks after your last period, when you may have just realized you are pregnant, it's important to get blood glucose under control before getting pregnant.

If blood glucose levels are kept near normal from the time of conception, the risk of birth defects in your baby can be greatly reduced to no higher than that of a women without diabetes. Unfortunately, more than half of the women with diabetes who become pregnant have unplanned pregnancies. It is critical if you have diabetes to be vigilant about blood glucose control when there is a possibility you might become pregnant. It is also critical that you use a reliable family planning method (see chapter 2), and that you don't stop using that method until your blood glucose levels are in your target range.

Because the increased blood glucose of most women who develop gestational diabetes develops during the second and third trimesters, the risk of the baby of a woman who has gestational diabetes developing birth defects is almost the same as that of a woman who does not have any type of diabetes, i.e., 1–4%.

There are, however, risks for both the mother and the child if you have gestational diabetes and your blood glucose levels are not controlled, or if you have type 1 or type 2 diabetes and your blood glucose levels are high after the first trimester. During the second and third trimesters, elevated blood glucose levels may contribute to the baby growing excessively. A big baby poses a risk to both mother and child. A woman who has diabetes, particularly one whose baby is large, may be more likely to have a difficult birth or to need a cesarean delivery. Compared with a woman who does not have diabetes and has a cesarean delivery, the woman who has diabetes is at increased risk of wound complications and infections following her cesarean. Risks for preterm delivery, low blood glucose, and serious respiratory problems in newborns are also higher when diabetes is poorly controlled in the last half of pregnancy.

As well as their babies being at risk, mothers who have gestational diabetes or diabetes that existed prior to pregnancy are at increased risk of certain medical problems, such as preeclampsia, a condition of pregnancy that causes high blood pressure and protein in the urine. Preeclampsia occasionally can progress to a more severe condition called eclampsia, in which seizures can occur. Preeclampsia may require bed rest, medications, and close follow-up for the mother until delivery. Because it is a potentially life-threatening disease, and because it does not go away until the baby is delivered, preeclampsia will probably require delivery before labor starts by itself.

Women with gestational diabetes are also at increased risk of developing diabetes after pregnancy. Work with your health care team to create a plan for managing blood glucose levels throughout your pregnancy to keep you and your baby healthy. If you have pre-existing diabetes or have had gestational diabetes in a previous pregnancy, chapter 2 will help you plan and prepare for pregnancy.

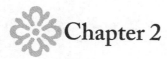 Chapter 2

Planning and Preparing for Pregnancy

Starting a family is one of the most important and life-changing steps in our lives. Preparing for pregnancy can help reduce preventable risks and help ensure a healthy pregnancy and a healthy start in life for your baby. If you have diabetes, controlling blood glucose levels prior to pregnancy greatly reduces the risk of birth defects.

Health and lifestyle choices affect the pregnancy and the development of your baby. Since almost half of pregnancies are unplanned, it is important to develop healthy habits and lifestyle choices before a pregnancy begins. Creating a reproductive health plan helps you set personal health goals so that you are emotionally, physically, and socially prepared.

Planning ahead permits you to establish a set of healthy lifestyle habits that will reduce the risk of complications and improve the health of your baby. This could be anything from achieving a healthy weight, eating better, and getting more physical activity, to cutting out alcohol or tobacco or altering any medications you may be on.

Review with your doctor any current or past health or social problems, the medications you use and whether they may affect the pregnancy, your genetic and family history, whether you are up to date on vaccinations, and any prior pregnancy complications. Also, discuss with your doctor any history or current use of alcohol, tobacco, or illicit substances. You may want to get help quitting as it is recommended that pregnant women and those attempting pregnancy should not smoke, drink, or use illicit substances, both to maintain their health and to prevent damage to their babies. Work with your health care providers to take charge of your health *before* trying to get pregnant.

Pregnancy Planning

If you have type 1 or type 2 you may benefit from a pre-pregnancy planning program. Your health care team can work with you to help you understand the importance of keeping your blood glucose levels in a target range both before and during pregnancy, potential risks for you and your baby, benefits of genetic counseling, and advice about family planning methods. You can also work with a diabetes nurse educator and a registered dietitian to outline a plan for achieving your target blood glucose goals. This plan will include an insulin regimen, nutritional management, physical activity, and frequent monitoring of blood glucose levels. Planning ahead is the best way to ensure that both you and your baby are as healthy as possible.

Family Planning and Family Spacing

There are certain steps you can take to prepare for a healthy pregnancy. First, ask yourself some important questions, including: how many children would you like to have and how many years would you like to have between children? If you are sexually active, do you have a plan to prevent pregnancy until you are ready? Having answers for these basic questions helps in the development of your reproductive health plan.

Women with diabetes have the same birth control options as women without diabetes. The pill, the intrauterine device (IUD), implants, barrier methods such as a diaphragm or condoms, and spermicides are all ways to reduce the risk of unplanned pregnancy. If you are sexually active and not emotionally or physically ready for pregnancy and parenting, using contraception (birth control) is of utmost importance. Which method you choose will depend on your own health history and you and your partner's preferences. If you have any concerns, be sure to bring them up with your health care team.

There are many methods of birth control, and all women with diabetes can find one that is safe and effective. However, if you also have other medical problems, such as kidney or heart disease, you may not be eligible to use estrogen-containing methods, such as the birth control pill, patch, or ring. Some pills do not have the hormone estrogen; however, these pills need to be taken at the same time every day or they are not as effective.

Birth control methods are best described by effectiveness, or how well they work at preventing pregnancy. The most effective methods are those with failure rates of <1%, meaning that less than 10 in 1,000 sexually active women will become pregnant per year using them.

HORMONAL CONTRACEPTIVES

Oral contraception, or birth control pills, are among the most popular and effective birth control methods available, about 95–99% effective. The pill refers to a variety of oral contraceptives that contain two synthetic hormones: estrogen and progesterone. Hormonal methods of birth control prevent pregnancy by preventing ovulation. Some pills contain both estrogen and progesterone, while others contain only progesterone.

Other types of hormonal contraceptives available are patches, vaginal rings, and by injection. The patch contains both estrogen and progesterone. You leave it on your skin for 21 days and then remove it for a week. The vaginal ring is a small circular device that also contains estrogen and progesterone. You insert it into your vagina and leave it there for 21 days every month. An injection called Depo-Provera contains only progesterone and is given at your doctor's office every three months.

In general, hormonal methods of birth control are safe for women with diabetes. Some women find that oral contraceptives cause their blood glucose to rise because of increased insulin resistance. If your blood glucose levels are affected, your insulin or oral medications can be adjusted. Make sure to check your blood glucose levels frequently, especially during the first few months of use.

There are also a few risk factors that can make these forms of birth control unsafe for you: if you are a smoker, or if you have a history of heart disease, stroke, high blood pressure, peripheral blood vessel disease, or blood clots. So talk to your doctor about your risk factors before starting hormonal contraceptives.

INTRAUTERINE DEVICES

Most women with diabetes are candidates for intrauterine devices (IUD). An IUD is a small device that is placed in the uterus during an outpatient visit by a health care provider. Some IUDs release the hormone progesterone into the uterus. IUDs prevent sperm from entering the egg and implanting in the uterus. IUDs can stay in place for one, five, or 10 years depending on the type, and can be removed at any time. IUDs work well for women with diabetes because they are extremely effective (95–98% effective) and do not affect medication needs or glucose control.

A visit to a physician is required for removal of an IUD, giving you an opportunity to optimize your health prior to attempting pregnancy. Your body is capable of getting pregnant as soon as the IUD is removed.

BARRIER METHODS

Barrier methods are another form of birth control that does not contain hormones, so they won't have an effect on blood glucose levels in women with diabetes. They are, however, less effective than other methods. Depending on the type, their effectiveness ranges from 74–94% in preventing pregnancy. Barrier methods include: condoms, diaphragm, sponge, cervical cap, and female condoms.

Condoms are excellent at preventing sexually transmitted diseases but are only 85% effective at preventing pregnancy. Given 1,000 sexually active women using only condoms for birth control, 150 of them will become pregnant within 1 year. Female condoms are a larger type of condom that you insert in your vagina up to 8 hours before intercourse. It is also effective at preventing sexually transmitted diseases. However, they are 74–79% effective in preventing pregnancy.

A diaphragm is a shallow rubber cup that fits over the cervix—the entrance to the uterus at the top of your vagina. It prevents sperm from entering the uterus. A diaphragm is 80–94% effective in preventing pregnancy. The effectiveness depends on your ability to place the device correctly. Your health care provider can teach you how to place it properly. It is kept in place for at least 6 hours after intercourse before it is removed.

The sponge and cervical cap also fit over the cervix to prevent sperm from entering the uterus. Both of these methods are 80–90% effective.

STERILIZATION

If you are not interested in having children now or in the future, there are several methods of permanent birth control. Vasectomy and female tubal sterilization should only be considered if you do not desire any more children. Vasectomy (men) is extremely safe but requires a cooperative partner. Tubal sterilization (women) is also safe, but comes with slightly increased risk of post-operative infection, along with the risks of general anesthesia. A tubal occlusion procedure may be done in the office as an outpatient and is also permanent. These methods are nearly 100% effective in preventing pregnancy. You should be certain about your decision to sterilize because it is quite complicated and sometimes impossible to reverse.

EMERGENCY CONTRACEPTION

Because birth control may fail (i.e., if a condom breaks or you forget to take your pill), there is a birth control option called emergency contraception that you can take as soon as possible within 120 hours (5 days) of unprotected sex. Emergency contraception prevents pregnancy most efficiently when taken within 72 hours (3 days) of having sex. It is about 85% effective at preventing pregnancy. Unless you have an allergy to the medication, there are no side effects to using this medication. You should not use this medication if you know that you are pregnant because it will not disrupt an existing pregnancy. It is available in pharmacies without a prescription to men and women over 17 years old. Those under 17 years old may obtain emergency contraception with a prescription. Some health care and family planning agencies supply both the prescription and emergency contraception for women below the age of 17. Many insurance plans will cover emergency contraception with a prescription for women of any age. It is recommended to use this for emergencies and not as your ongoing method of birth control because other methods of contraception are more effective if taken on a regular basis.

IF YOU ARE PREGNANT UNEXPECTEDLY

Despite your best efforts at using a family planning method, unexpected and unplanned pregnancies occur. If you find yourself unexpectedly pregnant, you may choose to continue the pregnancy and choose to parent, continue the pregnancy and choose adoption, or terminate the pregnancy (medical or surgical abortion). You should have an honest conversation with your health care provider about the risk or presence of birth defects and risks to your health so that this can help guide your decision regarding pregnancy options. If you choose to continue a pregnancy, you should seek medical attention immediately, especially if you have elevated blood glucose levels, to reduce the risk of elevated glucose levels doing harm to the developing baby.

Preparing for Pregnancy

Making the decision to start a family is an exciting time. Planning ahead permits you to establish a set of healthy lifestyle habits that will reduce the risk of complications and improve the health of your baby. For women with diabetes, this means an A1C as normal as possible (<7%), achieving or maintaining a healthy body weight, improving diet and exercise, and having a pre-pregnancy exam. This exam can help assess any problems that could jeopardize your health or your baby's health.

Your doctor may want you to make sure your A1C is less than 7 percent

Pre-Pregnancy Exam

Women with diabetes who are contemplating pregnancy should have a pre-pregnancy exam by their health care provider or specialist. This exam typically includes:

▶ Measuring your A1C level to make sure blood glucose levels are under control.

▶ An assessment of any complications, such as high blood pressure, heart disease, and kidney, nerve, and eye damage (eye doctor).

▶ Checking the function of your thyroid (if you have type 1 diabetes).

▶ Reviewing all your medications and supplements to make sure they are safe to continue using with pregnancy. Drugs commonly used to treat diabetes and its complications may not be recommended in pregnancy, especially statins, ACE inhibitors, ARBs, and most noninsulin therapies.

before you conceive. Doing so can prevent birth defects and infant death. A study of nearly 1,000 women found that the risk of infant death and birth defects increased as A1C topped 7 percent. When A1C, an estimate of average blood glucose levels over the past two to three months, was between 8.9 and 10.3, the women's risk doubled compared with a group of women without diabetes. Above 10.3, the women were four times as likely to have a poor outcome. Talk to your health care providers about your A1C goals before and during pregnancy.

Managing Blood Glucose

Women with diabetes have a higher risk of birth defects than women without diabetes; however, by keeping their blood glucose levels on target, they can lower their risks to the same level as women without diabetes (1–4%). This means keeping blood glucose levels as close to normal as possible before and during the first trimester of your pregnancy. All of your baby's major organs are formed during the first 6–8 weeks of your pregnancy, so managing your blood glucose levels before pregnancy is one of the most important factors for your pregnancy.

Some of the other problems that high blood glucose levels (hyperglycemia) may cause or contribute to are:

Risks for the mother
▶ Worsening of diabetic eye problems
▶ Worsening of diabetic kidney problems
▶ Infections of the urinary bladder and vaginal area
▶ Preeclampsia (high blood pressure usually with protein in the urine, which may develop during pregnancy)
▶ Difficult delivery or cesarean section

Risks for the baby
▶ Premature delivery
▶ Miscarriage
▶ Birth defects*
▶ Macrosomia (a big baby)
▶ Possibility of shoulder injury or nerve damage to the arm especially if a big baby is delivered vaginally

- Stillbirth
- Low blood glucose at birth (hypoglycemia)
- Prolonged jaundice (a yellow color to the skin)
- Respiratory distress syndrome (difficulty breathing)
- Twitching of the hands and feet, or cramping muscles caused by low calcium and magnesium levels.
  Not usually a risk for women with gestational diabetes.

In order to get your blood glucose levels under control, you may need to make some changes to your daily diabetes care. If you have type 1 diabetes, you might fine-tune your plan by increasing the number of injections you take each day or you may switch to insulin pump therapy (see chapter 4). You may need to monitor your blood glucose more frequently so that you can get good control without having too much hypoglycemia (low blood glucose). If you have type 2 diabetes and are currently using oral medications, your health care provider will probably have you switch to using insulin before and during your pregnancy (oral medications are unlikely to sufficiently lower your blood glucose to the levels needed for pregnancy).

Talk to your health care team about how to personalize your treatment plan and blood glucose target ranges for your health and your lifestyle.

Target Blood Glucose Goals Before Getting Pregnant

Premeal (before eating):   60–119 mg/dl

1 hour after meals: 100–149 mg/dl

Your health care provider may have you use goals such as these, but check with your own team about your specific goals. (*Managing Preexisting Diabetes and Pregnancy*, ADA, 2008)

Achieving a Healthy Body Weight

Achieving a healthy body weight before you become pregnant will make your pregnancy easier. Women who are underweight when they become pregnant are at increased risk of having a premature baby or having a baby born too small. Women who are overweight or obese when they become pregnant tend to have more complications during pregnancy (gestational diabetes or high blood pressure), prolonged, difficult labors, and a baby who weighs more than average. Their babies are more likely to have weight problems as adults that can also lead to chronic disease like diabetes and heart disease.

The first step in achieving a healthy pregnancy is to determine your healthy body weight. Healthy weight is defined by your body mass index (BMI), which is a ratio of your weight divided by your height squared, with weight measured in kilograms and height in meters. Your BMI level will show if you are underweight, in a normal weight range, overweight, or obese. You can calculate your BMI by using the BMI calculator at http://www.diabetes.org/food-and-fitness/fitness/weight-loss/bmi-calculator.html.

UNDERWEIGHT WOMEN

It is usually easier to gain than to lose weight; however, women with active athletic lifestyles or eating disorders may find it difficult to gain weight. Gaining some weight can improve fertility and may enable you to adjust your food intake to maintain a healthy rate of weight gain during pregnancy. Instead of focusing on weight gain, think about gradually increasing the amount of food you eat. If you are an athlete and have irregular or absent periods, talk to your health care team about adjusting your exercise regimen to allow for fertility.

OVERWEIGHT AND OBESE WOMEN

Being overweight can have a serious effect on reproduction as well as increase the risk of chronic disease. Overweight women are more likely to have fertility problems and abnormal periods. Losing about 10 percent of your body weight at a slow, gradual rate of no more than 1 pound/week is an appropriate goal for overweight women. Achieving this goal before you get pregnant will ensure that you have a healthier pregnancy. If you lose a few pounds before pregnancy, but you are still outside the normal range, don't despair. A minor weight loss can have a positive impact on your baby's health. Plus, small, gradual losses are easier to maintain over time.

If you are using certain oral medications or insulin to control your blood glucose, you may find that, as you lose weight, your blood glucose may occasionally fall to low levels. This is referred to as hypoglycemia (see chapter 4), and may or may not be associated with such symptoms as shakiness, nervousness, sweating, and a numb feeling around the mouth. Whether or not you have these symptoms when your blood glucose is low (less than 70 mg/dl) it is important to contact a member of your diabetes care team. You may be asked to lower your medication dose, change your activity, or make other adjustments to your daily activities.

BARIATRIC SURGERY BEFORE PREGNANCY

As obesity rates continue to rise, more and more women have elected to have bariatric surgery before pregnancy. Gastric banding and gastric bypass are the two types of surgeries. Studies suggest that pregnancy after bariatric surgery is safer than being pregnant as an extremely obese woman, as long as weight loss has stabilized before conception. Women who have had bariatric surgery should receive prenatal care from a team of specialists, including a high-risk obstetrician, a dietitian, and their bariatric surgeon.

Bariatric surgery can help you achieve a healthy weight, but it is not a quick fix. It requires significant changes in your lifestyle. Your medications may need to be taken in different forms, as they may not be absorbed effectively after some types of bariatric surgery.

Good nutrition is the key to having a healthy pregnancy following bariatric surgery. Vitamin and mineral supplementation is also important as your body will absorb less of these nutrients after this surgery. You will need to take these supplements indefinitely from the time of your operation. Supplementing good food sources with a once-a-day vitamin/mineral supplement will help assure a healthy pregnancy. It is also important for pregnant women who have had bariatric surgery to be mindful of food choices and portion sizes during pregnancy to prevent regaining the weight they've just lost. Regular exercise will also help keep your weight gain during pregnancy within an appropriate range.

Your weight loss will occur over a 6–12-month period. If you decide to have gastric bypass surgery, you should delay your next pregnancy until you have reached a steady weight (usually after at least 18 months). Gastric banding causes a more gradual loss of weight and has a smaller effect on nutrition. Women who have gastric banding surgery should wait at least 6 months to conceive.

For those patients who need and choose bariatric surgery and achieve a BMI less than 30, the good news is that the health benefits are significant. Women who have undergone this surgery have lower risks of high blood pressure, diabetes, and infertility. They may also find that their existing medical complications become easier to manage or even, in some cases, completely disappear.

Improving Diet and Exercise Habits

Healthy eating and regular exercise are key lifestyle habits that improve your health and set the course for a healthy pregnancy and for the rest of your life. If you are planning a pregnancy, you want your baby to be as healthy as possible. The best way to do this is to make yourself as healthy as possible. Incorporating healthy eating and moderate exercise into your life is a great start. The table below will give you a good idea of some basic components to a healthy meal plan. You can find more information about healthy eating and exercise during pregnancy in chapter 6.

Along with eating nutritious food, getting the proper vitamins and minerals is also important to your pre-pregnancy health. Iron and folic acid are two nutrients that play an important role in the growth and development of your baby.

Folic acid is the only nutrient supplement recommended for women planning pregnancies because it is important for preventing birth defects of the brain and spinal cord. For this reason, it is recommended that you start supplementing with folic acid *before* you become pregnant. The federal government currently requires flour and breakfast cereals to be fortified to raise the folic acid intake of Americans. However, this may not be a sufficient amount to prevent certain kinds of birth defects called neural tube defects. It is recommended that women of child-bearing age take an additional 600 micrograms of folic acid daily either separately or as part of a multivitamin supplement. It is also wise to increase your intake of folic acid–rich foods (spinach, romaine lettuce, wheat germ, fortified breakfast cereals, legumes). Check with your health care provider to find out how much folic acid you should incorporate into your diet and take as a supplement before pregnancy.

You probably won't need to take an iron supplement before pregnancy, unless your doctor recommends it to overcome a deficiency, but you should try to eat at least two servings of iron-rich foods daily. Iron in animal products (such as beef, pork, lamb, or poultry) is absorbed most easily, but you can also get iron from plant foods (dark green vegetables, or legumes—for example, lentils, beans, chickpeas, soybeans, tofu). Iron deficiency is the most common nutritional deficiency in the United States. It is a particular problem among pregnant women because more iron is needed throughout pregnancy to expand your blood volume and for your baby's growth. For this reason, prenatal vitamins usually contain iron.

Regular physical activity is another essential component of a healthy lifestyle. Exercise helps control body weight, control blood glucose, improve mood, and reduce the risk of cardiovascular disease. Achieving a regular exercise pattern before pregnancy will help you begin your pregnancy at a healthier body weight. Aim for at least 30 minutes of physical activity most, if not all, days of the week. You can read more about continuing physical activity during pregnancy in chapter 6.

Health Goals During Pregnancy

It's important to set your own goals and follow through on them. Remember that any changes you make to make yourself healthier will also impact the health of your baby during your pregnancy.

▶ Set goals to get six to eight hours of sleep each night.

▶ Eat plenty of fresh fruit, vegetables, and whole grains daily, and decrease the intake of saturated and trans fats in your daily diet.

▶ Cut out alcohol, tobacco, or illicit drug use as soon as possible because these can all have a negative effect on your child's development.

▶ Have regular doctor, eye doctor, and dental checkups. Make sure you have any health problems under control, or work with your doctor to develop a plan of care.

▶ Be physically active at least 30 minutes 5 days a week.

Chapter 3

Special Care During Pregnancy

Congratulations, you're pregnant! Your pregnancy is one of the most important times to take good care of yourself and your diabetes. This chapter focuses on the stages of pregnancy, your health care team (who will help you manage your health and deal with any special circumstances), tests you can expect during pregnancy, possible complications, and the importance of a support system.

The Stages of Pregnancy

Pregnancy lasts about nine months, or 40 weeks, and is divided into trimesters. By dividing your pregnancy into three different time periods, it is easier for your health care team to monitor the growth of the baby over the pregnancy.

THE FIRST TRIMESTER

During the first few weeks, your baby's heart forms and begins pumping blood. The digestive system, backbone, spinal cord, and brain begin to form. The placenta also develops at this time. The placenta is the organ that connects you with your baby. It provides a filtering system to allow nutrients to pass into the baby's bloodstream from yours. The placenta also makes hormones needed to keep you and your baby healthy during pregnancy.

Around the eighth week of pregnancy, your baby will develop eyes (with the lids still joined closed at first), nose, lips, and tongue. Arms, elbows, forearms, hands, knees, lower legs, and feet begin to form. Before the ninth week, your baby is technically known as an embryo. However, after the ninth week, it is called a fetus.

By the end of the first trimester, your baby will be about 3 inches long and weigh about 1 1/2 ounces. The buds and sockets of teeth in the jawbones begin to form. Fingernails and toenails start to develop. The earlobes are formed and your baby will have most of her or his organs and tissues.

THE SECOND TRIMESTER

Your baby continues to grow and develop during the second trimester. About a month into the second trimester (4 months along) your baby will weigh about 7 ounces and will be 6 to 7 inches long. At the beginning of this trimester, your baby's heartbeat will become audible and you may be able to hear it with either your doctor's stethoscope or the Doppler device that amplifies the baby's heartbeat. The baby's muscles and bones are formed. Hair grows on the head and eyebrows begin to appear. By 20 weeks, you may even be able to feel the baby move.

Near the end of the second trimester (6 months), the baby will weigh close to 1¾ pounds and might be 11 to 14 inches long. You will notice your baby's movements more often. The eyelids will separate and eyelashes will form. Also, the fingernails grow to the ends of the baby's fingers.

THE THIRD TRIMESTER

All vital organs are fully formed. The baby's head bones are soft and flexible. Your baby will now begin to gain weight and grow rapidly. By the end of the seventh month, your baby will weigh 2 1/2 to 3 pounds and be 11 to 14 inches long. By the time your baby is ready to be delivered, he or she will weigh about 7 to 8 1/2 pounds and be close to 20 inches long.

Your Health Care Team

During your pregnancy, you will see different members of a health care team who are specially trained to care for pregnant women with diabetes. It's important to remember that YOU are the leader of this team. Besides yourself, this team usually consists of an obstetrician, a diabetes care provider, a diabetes educator, and a dietitian.

Obstetricians are physicians who will look after your pregnancy, monitor your health, watch the growth of your baby, and deliver the baby. If you had diabetes before pregnancy, your obstetrician, who may be a specialist in high-risk pregnancies (perinatologist), will see you every 4 weeks initially, and more often as the pregnancy progresses. You may see your physician weekly during the last month of pregnancy. It is wise to also prepare to have a pediatrician who is experienced in the care of infants of mothers with diabetes once the baby is born.

Your diabetes care provider will help you look after your blood glucose control during your pregnancy. This care provider can be an endocrinologist, primary care physician, or obstetrician. You will probably also see a diabetes nurse educator with specialization in teaching women how to intensively manage their diabetes during pregnancy.

You should also start seeing a dietitian who can help you prepare a meal plan and make sure you're getting the necessary nutrition to keep you and your baby healthy during pregnancy. If you were not already doing these things, you will likely learn how to count carbohydrates and adjust insulin doses based on your carb intake and blood glucose patterns.

Tests to Expect During Pregnancy

Now that you're familiar with your health care team, let's take a look at the tests you can expect during pregnancy. Most of these tests are standard for all pregnant women and are nothing to be afraid of. Just remember: all of them are in place to help ensure you have the healthiest baby possible. Discuss any questions you have with your health care team to alleviate any stress you may have about the procedures.

The first test you will likely have during pregnancy is a test to confirm that you are indeed pregnant. This will be either a urine or blood test.

After the pregnancy has been confirmed, your caregiver will probably send you for an ultrasound examination. In the second half of the pregnancy you may have additional ultrasound examinations to estimate the baby's growth as well as the amount of amniotic fluid that surrounds the baby.

ULTRASOUND

Ultrasound examinations (also called scans or sonograms) are a routine part of most pregnancies. The ultrasound examination is your first chance to look at your baby. The first ultrasound you will have will likely be performed in the first trimester of pregnancy. This ultrasound is known as the "dating ultrasound," because it will tell you the estimated due date and how far along you are (weeks pregnant). The earlier in pregnancy the baby is measured, the more accurate the dating. It will also tell you if there is more than one baby in your uterus.

The ultrasound machine uses very high frequency sound waves (so high that they cannot be heard by the human ear) that are sent through a hand-held instrument called a transducer. The technician or doctor will move the transducer over your abdomen and your baby will appear on the monitor. Early in pregnancy, it might be done when you have a full bladder, so that your uterus can be seen. Sometimes early in pregnancy your doctor may perform the ultrasound by inserting the transducer into your vagina. The information collected by the transducer is then turned into two- or three-dimensional pictures of the baby (or babies) on a computer screen. Ultrasound has been found to be very safe for the baby, even when performed many times during the pregnancy.

After this ultrasound examination your physician will be able to tell you your estimated due date even if your periods were not regular before the pregnancy. Having an accurate due date is very important because many of the decisions regarding the management of your pregnancy depend on this information. The earlier in pregnancy an ultrasound examination is performed, the more accurate the estimated delivery date will be. An ultrasound is often repeated at one- to three-month intervals to monitor the growth of the baby.

SCREENING TESTS FOR DOWN SYNDROME

Some women choose to have screening for Down syndrome performed during the first half of their pregnancies. Down syndrome is a genetic condition where a person has 47 chromosomes instead of the usual 46. Physical, mental, and social development is often delayed. Women with diabetes do not have a higher risk of having a baby with Down syndrome, but older women do.

There are many different methods to screen for Down syndrome and your caregiver will explain them to you at one of your first visits. If you choose to undergo screening for Down syndrome, it's important to remember that even if the test comes back positive, it only means that your risk of Down syndrome is higher. Approximately 3–5 women out of 100 test positive during the screening, but most of them do not have a baby with Down syndrome.

If the screening blood and/or ultrasound test is positive, a specialized ultrasound may be done. The definite test to determine whether the baby has Down syndrome is an amniocentesis. This test involves using ultrasound to guide a needle through your abdomen into the fluid that surrounds the baby. This fluid contains cells from the baby that can be tested for Down syndrome as well as for problems with other chromosomes. Before you decide whether to have this test your caregiver will discuss the possible risks associated with the amniocentesis and might also send you for a consultation with a genetic specialist.

THE "ANATOMY" SCAN

Between 18 and 20 weeks (and sometimes earlier) a detailed ultrasound scan of your baby is offered. At this time, the baby is usually large enough for all the distinct features to show up on the test. You may find out the sex of your baby during this ultrasound, though sex determinations are not always accurate.

The main purpose of the ultrasound is to examine the baby to rule out any major birth defects. Women with type 1 or type 2 diabetes whose glucose levels were not well controlled when they became pregnant have a higher risk of their baby having a birth defect. Luckily, most of these problems can be found on this detailed ultrasound examination.

Two of the birth defects that are more common in women with type

1 or 2 diabetes whose glucose levels haven't been controlled well are heart defects and spina bifida. Spina bifida is a birth defect in which the backbone and spinal canal do not close before birth, leaving the spinal cord exposed.

You may also be offered an extra ultrasound of the baby's heart called a "fetal echocardiogram." This ultrasound is usually performed by either a pediatric cardiologist or a high-risk pregnancy specialist and is usually performed toward the middle or later part of the second trimester, when the baby's heart is big enough to see its details.

TESTS OF PLACENTAL FUNCTION

The placenta is the organ that develops inside your uterus during pregnancy and transmits the nutrients and oxygen to your baby needed for development. Placental function is sometimes affected in type 1 and type 2 diabetes, especially if you have retinopathy (eye disease) or nephropathy (kidney disease). Blood tests, ultrasound, or Doppler blood flow measurements can be used to test the placenta's function and make sure your baby is receiving the blood and nutrients that he/she needs. Doppler measures the way blood flows in different blood vessels inside the baby and the uterus. Recent studies have shown that collecting this information might help predict your risk of developing complications related to the function of the placenta later in pregnancy.

FETAL WELL-BEING TESTS

There are several tests throughout the second half of your pregnancy that your doctor might recommend to check on the health, growth rate, and general well-being of your baby. These include the kick count test, biophysical profile test (BPP), non-stress test, and contraction stress test. Talk to your doctor about which tests are recommended for you.

The kick count test is the most common test and can be done at 20 weeks. It simply involves counting the time it takes to feel 10 kicks or movements by the baby. This should happen within two hours, and will often happen in less time. Every baby has different movement patterns. It's also important to remember that babies sleep, so there may be times when he/she isn't moving. To perform this test, lie on your side and count the movements over a two-hour period. If you aren't feeling enough movement, try again in an hour or two. If the baby still isn't moving enough, contact your health care provider. It's also a good idea to contact your caregiver if you notice a sudden decrease in the baby's movements compared to what you normally experience. Kick counting is typically done between weeks 32–40.

Another test that's used to check on the well-being of the baby is the biophysical profile (BPP). The BPP is an ultrasound examination that looks at the baby's body movements, body tone, breathing movements, and amount of amniotic fluid in the uterus, along with a nonstress test (see below). The BPP is performed more often in women with type 1 and 2 diabetes. This test is typically done between weeks 34–40.

A "nonstress test" (NST) monitors the baby's heart rate non-invasively. The test involves attaching one device to a belt on the mother's abdomen to measure the baby's heart rate and another device attached to a belt to measure contractions. Fetal movement, heart rate, and heart rate patterns are measured for 20–30 minutes. Often the results of an NST are followed by a BPP and the results are combined. This test is typically done between weeks 34–40.

A contraction stress test (CST) is a test that is used less commonly and that is very similar to the NST but will check your baby's response to contractions of your uterus.

If your baby is to be delivered before 39 weeks your doctor might perform an amniocentesis. This test is performed by inserting a special needle into your uterus, then drawing out a bit of the fluid surrounding your baby and sending it for tests to determine if the baby's lungs have matured. This test is usually done only if there is uncertainty regarding your due date, and/or if it appears that it would be safest to deliver your baby before (s)he is due.

Diabetes Complications During Pregnancy

It is possible for diabetes complications to develop or worsen during pregnancy in women with diabetes diagnosed before pregnancy (type 1 or type 2 diabetes). Understanding your risks for complications helps you to be alert for any signs and symptoms of complications. This does not apply to women with gestational diabetes, as most such women should not have any special problems related to diabetes during pregnancy.

As with all diabetes complications, keeping your blood glucose levels in your target range (see chapter 4) is the best way to prevent or delay complications. The less time you spend with high blood glucose levels, the lower your risk for developing diabetes complications. Even if you already have complications, it's not too late to slow the progression. Lowering blood glucose levels can help you improve most complications—even if they've already developed.

EYE DISEASE (RETINOPATHY)

Retinopathy is damage to small blood vessels in the eye that can lead to vision problems. Diabetes eye disease can worsen during pregnancy. If you had eye disease before the pregnancy, have had poor blood glucose control, or have difficulty controlling your blood pressure, you are at risk of worsening eye disease during pregnancy.

If you had no eye disease before the pregnancy, your chance of developing eye disease in the pregnancy is small, and if eye disease does develop, it is likely it will go away after the pregnancy. Women with diabetes should be seen by an eye care specialist in the first trimester of pregnancy. The eye care specialist will decide if more visits during pregnancy or postpartum are needed. If you have severe eye disease that needs to be treated with laser therapy, it is safe to receive this treatment during pregnancy.

There is no evidence that women who become pregnant have more eye disease in the long term than women who don't become pregnant.

NEUROPATHY

Neuropathy is a disease of the nervous system. If you have damage to the nerves that control heart rate or blood pressure, it can affect how you will respond to the physical stresses of pregnancy. Neuropathy of the stomach (gastroparesis) or intestines can affect how well your body nourishes you and your growing baby. Tell your health care provider if you have a history of gastroparesis or if you have persistent problems with nausea, vomiting, or diarrhea.

KIDNEY DISEASE (NEPHROPATHY)

Nephropathy is disease of the kidneys. Hyperglycemia (chapter 4) and high blood pressure can damage the kidneys. Nephropathy from diabetes can be mild, in which case the kidneys still function normally and the only sign is small amounts of protein in the urine (called microalbuminuria). Nephropathy that is more severe causes reduced kidney function. Nephropathy can worsen during pregnancy. If you have protein in the urine, this will probably increase during pregnancy, but it will go back to pre-pregnancy levels after you have your baby, and the chance of more severe kidney disease is not worsened by pregnancy. If you have more advanced kidney disease before you get pregnant, there is some risk of your kidney function worsening during the pregnancy. Some swelling, particularly of the face, feet, and ankles, can be a normal part of being pregnant. Excessive swelling of the ankles, as well as puffy hands and face, occur with kidney disease. Therefore, during pregnancy, swelling by itself is not a reliable sign that kidney disease is either developing or getting worse. Your care providers should monitor your kidney function carefully with blood and urine tests.

Women with kidney disease from diabetes often have high blood pressure that may also worsen during pregnancy. If you have kidney disease from diabetes you are at higher risk of developing complications in the pregnancy, such as preeclampsia (sudden worsening of blood pressure, often with worsening protein in the urine), delivering your baby early, or having a small baby. For the best outcomes possible, women and their caregivers should aim for excellent blood glucose control and excellent blood pressure control.

HIGH BLOOD PRESSURE (HYPERTENSION)

Women who have diabetes are at increased risk of developing high blood pressure. Your blood pressure will be checked throughout the pregnancy and, if necessary, pills to lower your blood pressure will be given to you. If you had high blood pressure before the pregnancy, your medications may need to be changed during the pregnancy. Some pills such as angiotensin-converting enzyme inhibitors (ACE-inhibitors) or angiotensin II receptor blockers (ARBs) are not recommended during pregnancy because they can cause problems for the baby. Consult your doctor at the earliest possible date to see if your medication needs to be changed.

If you had high blood pressure before the pregnancy, your chance of worsening blood pressure (preeclampsia) is higher than it is for other women. If you did not have high blood pressure before pregnancy but did have diabetes, your chance of developing preeclampsia is somewhat higher than a woman who does not have diabetes. Swelling of arms and legs commonly goes along with this condition, but swelling is a normal part of pregnancy. Preeclampsia can be dangerous for the mother and the baby and may require bed rest for the mother until delivery. Delivery is the only known effective treatment for preeclampsia. Fortunately, preeclampsia usually develops toward the end of the third trimester when the risks to your baby from preterm delivery are minimal.

HEART DISEASE (CARDIAC DISEASE)

If you have had diabetes for a long time you may be asked to undergo tests to check your heart, such as an ECG (electrocardiogram) and possibly a stress test (treadmill test). This is to make sure that you don't have heart disease that could affect your health and that of your baby during the pregnancy.

THYROID TESTS

If you have type 1 diabetes, you may be asked to have a blood test for thyroid function. Abnormal thyroid function is not uncommon in women with type 1 diabetes as they may have antibodies that act against their thyroid gland, making that gland produce too much or too little thyroid hormone. If you were on a pill to treat an underactive thyroid (levothyroxine) before getting pregnant, the dose may need to be adjusted after you get pregnant, due to the changes in hormones during pregnancy. If your thyroid is functioning abnormally during pregnancy your diabetes team may want to have an endocrinologist determine the appropriate treatment for you.

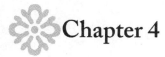

Chapter 4

Blood Glucose Control

Keeping your blood glucose levels as close to normal before and during pregnancy can help eliminate birth defects or complications associated with diabetes. You will need to check your blood glucose levels several times a day to prevent low blood glucose (hypoglycemia) or high blood glucose (hyperglycemia). Even with great care, you still may experience occasional problems with hypoglycemia and hyperglycemia. If you are taking insulin (see chapter 5), you may be asked to monitor your blood glucose levels before and after meals and at bedtime. If you have type 2 or gestational diabetes and are managing it through meal planning and regular exercise, you may need to check your blood glucose more frequently than usual. Most women with type 2 need to start insulin at some point during pregnancy to keep blood glucose levels in their target range.

During the first trimester of your pregnancy, blood glucose targets are designed to help you minimize the risk of birth defects and miscarriage. In the second and third trimesters, your glucose targets will help prevent your baby from getting too large. If you have trouble staying in your target range or have frequent low blood glucose levels, talk to your health care team about revising your treatment plan. Target blood glucose values for gestational, type 1, or type 2 diabetes may differ slightly in different care systems and with different diabetic teams. The box below contains blood glucose targets that are often used for pregnant women who require treatment with insulin. You and your health care team should discuss your personal target goals.

Sample Blood Glucose Targets Before and During Pregnancy

Target blood glucose values before and during early pregnancy

Before meals:	60–119 mg/dl
One hour after meals:	100–149 mg/dl
A1C:	less than 6%

Target blood glucose values during second and third trimesters of pregnancy

Before meals:	60–99 mg/dl
One hour after meals:	100–129 mg/dl
A1C:	less than 6%

Adapted from Managing Preexisting Diabetes and Pregnancy, *ADA, 2008.*

The factors that affect blood glucose levels include diet, exercise, weight gain, and medications. It is almost impossible to achieve good blood glucose control with diabetes without following a meal plan. Food raises your blood glucose levels. Carbohydrates are the foods that provide energy for the body but also raise your blood glucose the most. The best way to keep your blood glucose levels in the normal range is to be sure that the carbohydrates you eat are nutritious (for example, fruits and vegetables or whole grains rather than desserts or sodas), matching your insulin doses to the amount of carbohydrate you eat, and working with your dietitian to determine how much carbohydrate you should eat. More details about what, when, and how much to eat while pregnant may be found in chapter 6.

Exercise during pregnancy can help your body utilize blood glucose, and help control your weight gain. It can also prepare you for labor and childbirth and give you an overall feeling of well-being. Walking is one of the best exercises for pregnant women. Walking for 20–30 minutes after a meal, at least once a day, will help you to lower your blood glucose levels. There are other appropriate exercises for pregnant women, such as swimming, low-impact aerobics, and bicycling. Before starting any exercise program you should check with your obstetrician for his or her recommendations or restrictions. More information about exercise and pregnancy is in chapter 6.

How much weight you should gain will be determined based on your body weight and height as well as your baby's needs. During the first three months (the first trimester), weight gain is usually very little—probably only two to four pounds if you are of average weight. During the second trimester, you should gain weight at a much faster rate—about one pound per week if you are of average weight, and one-half pound per week if you are overweight or obese. More details about weight gain during pregnancy may be found in chapter 6.

Insulin is the traditional first-choice drug for glucose control during pregnancy. All women with type 1 diabetes need insulin, and most women with type 2 diabetes will need insulin during pregnancy. About 10% of women who have gestational diabetes and who start their treatment with diet and exercise alone will need insulin or some other medication added to their treatment to keep their blood glucose levels in control as their pregnancies advance. There are many types of insulin. Insulin is discussed in more detail in chapter 5.

Now that you know the factors that affect your blood glucose levels, it's time to talk about how to monitor your glucose levels on a day-to-day basis.

Blood Glucose Monitoring

Self-monitoring of blood glucose is the main tool used to check your day-to-day diabetes control. Monitoring allows you and your care team to better understand how diet, exercise, insulin, stress, and illness affect your blood glucose levels, so you can get the best diabetes control possible.

If your blood glucose levels are controlled by diet and exercise, you may be asked to test your blood glucose four times a day. Blood glucose checks are individually tailored to each woman and her pregnancy. Generally, tests are done before and/or after breakfast, lunch, and dinner, and at bedtime. The frequency of glucose testing may be reduced or increased according to your glucose control, or as needed to guide your care. Especially if you are using insulin or oral medications or have type 1 or type 2 diabetes, it may also be necessary to test at 2–3 a.m.

BLOOD GLUCOSE METERS

The best way to check your blood glucose is with a blood glucose meter. Blood glucose meters are small, computerized machines that "read" your blood glucose. Blood glucose meters use strips that do a chemical reaction with glucose in the blood. The meter "reads" the mix of chmicals and blood glucose on the strips and converts them to a small electric signal that depends on how much glucose is present. The meter reads the electric signal and converts it to a blood glucose reading, which shows on the screen as a number in milligrams per deciliter (mg/dl).

You now have more choices than ever when it comes to blood glucose meters. The main factors you will want to think about when choosing a meter are: cost (insurance coverage, price of test strips); performance (accuracy, batteries, and meter replacement); and suitability for your lifestyle (size, meter memory). Along with a meter you will also need lancets (small sterile pointed object used to prick the skin in order to obtain a drop of blood) and test strips. Blood will be placed on the test strip and inserted into the meter. Be sure your doctor or diabetes educator shows you the correct way to use your meter.

You can find the latest tools that will help you self-monitor your blood glucose levels during day-to-day life in the American Diabetes Association's magazine, *Diabetes Forecast*. This publication contains a Consumer Guide for patients in every January edition. It includes the latest blood glucose monitoring tools on the market. You can also find the consumer guide at http://forecast.diabetes.org/magazine/features/2011-consumer-guide.

Keeping a log of your blood glucose results will help you to note the effects of what you have eaten, as well as the effects of exercise and other special circumstances on your blood glucose. Most blood glucose meters on the market have an internal memory that can record glucose readings. It's important to still keep track on your own in case the meter's memory fails. You can do this in a log book, an online program, or even on new smartphone applications. Bringing your glucose meter and glucose log to all of your prenatal appointments will make it easier for your diabetes team to evaluate your glucose control.

CONTINUOUS GLUCOSE MONITORING

A recently new device on the market is the continuous glucose monitor

(CGM). There are currently four CGMs on the U.S. market. Like your blood glucose meter, it measures glucose levels; however, unlike a blood glucose meter, a CGM is attached to you and measures your glucose levels throughout the day. The device uses a sensor to measure interstitial glucose levels just under the skin. The sensor transmits the results to a handheld receiver or insulin pump every few minutes so you know what your glucose levels are throughout the day. This is helpful because it can help you catch spikes and dips you may have missed between tests with your meter. You can download the data and follow trends to better manage your diabetes.

CGMs aren't right for everyone. Many insurance companies won't cover CGMs for people with type 2 diabetes, so make sure to check with your insurance company first before shopping around. Talk to your health care team to see if a CGM might be a good option for you.

High Blood Glucose (Hyperglycemia)

Too much glucose in the blood is called hyperglycemia. High blood glucose levels over a prolonged period of time early in pregnancy may lead to birth defects. High blood glucose later in pregnancy may lead to premature delivery, having a large baby, and low blood glucose (hypoglycemia) in the baby following delivery. If you have gestational diabetes, hyperglycemia can lead to preeclampsia (high blood pressure and swelling) and urinary tract infections in you. Having a high blood glucose level during a single blood glucose check is not going to cause birth defects in your baby. These complications arise when your blood glucose levels are high for a prolonged amount of time. Checking your blood glucose levels frequently is the best way to know if your blood glucose levels are higher than your target range.

In women with pre-existing type 1 or type 2 diabetes, high blood glucose levels during the first 8 weeks of pregnancy can cause birth defects. Birth defects can affect the heart, spinal cord, brain, and bones.

Hyperglycemia can happen for several reasons. You may eat more than you planned or exercise less than planned. If you are on insulin, you may not have taken enough or your doses may need to be adjusted. Other things can cause hyperglycemia, such as the stress of an illness like a cold or the flu. Emotional stress, such as family or work conflicts, may also contribute to hyperglycemia. Finally, as pregnancy advances, the normal insulin resistance that occurs due to pregnancy-generated hormones progressively increases. This may be noticed most by women who have type 2 diabetes. Frequent adjustments to your insulin dose throughout pregnancy should help you to keep your blood glucose at levels that are safe for you and your unborn baby.

Signs and Symptoms of Hyperglycemia

High blood glucose may not have symptoms, but when more severe its symptoms may include:

▶ Blurry vision

▶ Hunger

▶ Upset stomach

▶ Frequent urination

▶ Dry, itchy skin

▶ Headaches

▶ Thirst

▶ Tiredness and fatigue

HOW TO TREAT HYPERGLYCEMIA

The best way to avoid hyperglycemia is to follow your meal plan and exercise regimen, and work with your care team to make sure your insulin doses are correct. It's also important to test your blood regularly and then treat high blood sugar early before it gets higher. Your doctor can tell you what levels are above your target range. Target blood glucose levels may be found on page 46.

There are three ways to lower blood glucose levels: exercise, eat less carbohydrate, or take more insulin. Your health care provider can help you to work out procedures for handling one-time hyperglycemia as well as more detailed instructions for handling patterns of high blood glucose. Also, discuss what level of blood glucose warrants an immediate call to the health care team.

DIABETIC KETOACIDOSIS

Ketones are made when your body burns stored fat for energy. Large amounts of ketones can harm you or your baby. In women with diabetes, the presence of ketones in the blood and urine may be a sign of a condition called ketoacidosis. Ketoacidosis is an emergency condition in which an insufficient amount of insulin is circulating in your blood. Glucose is the body's major source of energy. Certain cells in the body (especially muscle cells) need insulin to get glucose out of the blood and into these cells. When insulin is low or absent, blood glucose concentrations rise, but these important cells are deprived of glucose, their primary source of energy. The body responds by breaking down fats into ketones.

Ketones are acids that can cross into the glucose-starved cells and serve as an alternate source of energy when, because of the low insulin level, these cells cannot get enough glucose. Ketones are an inefficient source of energy. Too many ketones in the blood change the body chemistry of both mother and unborn baby, and may cause severe damage, up to and including death to one or both. Therefore, diabetic ketoacidosis must be treated immediately upon recognition. Signs of ketoacidosis are: nausea, vomiting, stomach pain, thirst, excessive urination, fruity odor on the breath, and rapid breathing.

Small amounts of ketones in the urine, particularly before breakfast, are not uncommon during pregnancy. Therefore, some diabetes experts do not recommend routine testing of urine ketones during pregnancy. It is important to discuss with your health care team if, when, and how often you should test for urine ketones, and what results should lead to a phone call or emergency room visit. Urine test strips are available at your local pharmacy without a prescription. One blood glucose meter also has an option to test blood ketones.

Low Blood Glucose (Hypoglycemia)

During pregnancy, blood glucose levels below 60 or 70 mg/dl are referred to as hypoglycemia. If you take insulin and keep your blood glucose levels near normal, you are more likely to have episodes of low blood glucose. There is no evidence that hypoglycemia is harmful for the baby, but a severe hypoglycemic event can be dangerous for the mother and baby, for example if it leads to a car accident. Hypoglycemia can occur due to taking too much insulin, skipping or delaying meals, or doing excessive exercise. The single most important way to prevent hypoglycemia is to test your blood glucose regularly. Glucose monitoring is the only way to know how your body responds to food, exercise, insulin, and stress. In addition to checking before and after physical activity, always check your blood glucose before you drive.

Some women, particularly those who have type 1 diabetes, may develop hypoglycemia unawareness during pregnancy. When this occurs, you may not experience early warning signs of hypoglycemia. You may have less sweating and shakiness and more rapid development of drowsiness and confusion. Because you may not experience symptoms of hypoglycemia, regular testing is necessary to detect hypoglycemia. Because hypoglycemia unawareness produces signs and symptoms that may be misinterpreted as mental illness or being on an illicit drug, it is a good idea to wear a bracelet or pendant that says that you have diabetes. These may be purchased in drug stores and online.

Talk to your health care team about the blood glucose level at which you should start treating hypoglycemia, and how to best treat it when and if it occurs.

Warning Signs of Hypoglycemia

▶ Clammy
▶ Sweaty
▶ Confused
▶ Pale
▶ Shaky or dizzy

▶ Tired
▶ Blurry vision
▶ Dry mouth
▶ Headache
▶ Pounding heart beat

HOW TO TREAT HYPOGLYCEMIA

You can treat low blood glucose by eating or drinking something that contains fast-acting carbohydrates (see Treating hypoglycemia, below). Always carry with you a form of fast-acting carbohydrate. The easiest form is found in glucose tablets—a chewable tablet made of pure glucose used to treat hypoglycemia. These are available without prescription in most pharmacies.

The most common recommendation for treating hypoglycemia is to follow the "rule of 15." If your blood glucose is low, consume 15 grams of carbohydrates, wait 15 minutes, and recheck your blood glucose level. If you still have low blood glucose, you may need to take another dose of 15 grams. Check again in 15 minutes, and repeat, if necessary. Having a glucagon kit at home and at work is a good idea in case of severe hypoglycemia, particularly for women with type 1 diabetes. Glucagon is a hormone that causes your blood glucose to rise. It is used primarily to treat someone who has passed out from hypoglycemia, or someone who is too confused to eat or drink. It is a good idea to teach family members and coworkers how and when to inject you with glucagon, just in case you have a severe reaction.

Treating Hypoglycemia

15 Grams of Fast-Acting Carbohydrate are found in:

▶ 3–4 glucose tablets (check ahead of time to see if each is 4 or 5 grams)

▶ 1 gel tube

▶ 2 tablespoons raisins

▶ 1/2 cup regular soda (not diet)

▶ 4 ounces orange juice

▶ 5–7 Lifesavers

▶ 6 jellybeans

▶ 3 teaspoons sugar, honey, or corn syrup

▶ 6–8 ounces nonfat or 1% milk

Blood glucose monitoring and treating low and high blood glucose during pregnancy are a huge part of you and your baby staying healthy if you have diabetes. Along with meal plans and exercise, insulin will probably be used to control your blood glucose levels. Read more about different insulin types, how insulin works, and how it's administered in the next chapter.

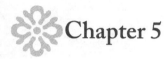

Chapter 5

Insulin and Other Medications

Insulin is the traditional first-choice drug for blood glucose control during pregnancy, because it is the most effective for fine-tuning blood glucose and it does not cross the placenta. All women with type 1 diabetes need insulin; women with type 2 are usually switched to insulin for pregnancy because the insulin resistance of pregnancy makes oral agents not work well enough to keep blood glucose levels in your target range. For women with gestational diabetes, meal planning and exercise often work to keep blood glucose levels in control; however, if blood glucose levels are still high, your doctor will probably start you on insulin. Insulin is more commonly used for gestational diabetes, but occasionally oral diabetes medications might be used. The four types of insulin in common use during pregnancy in the U.S. are: rapid-acting, regular, intermediate-acting, and long-acting insulin.

Insulin cannot be taken as a pill. It would have to be broken down like food before it could begin working. Insulin needs to be injected to work well. Insulin can be injected with a traditional syringe, an insulin pen, or through an insulin pump. All three methods are safe for pregnant women. Because insulin is naturally made in the body, insulin allergies are very rare. This makes it a very effective treatment option.

Usually the amount of insulin you take increases with each trimester. Some women need to increase their insulin dose by as much as two or three times, especially in the last trimester. You'll probably need more insulin throughout your pregnancy because the hormones of pregnancy, which increase over time, create more insulin resistance. So, if you have pre-existing type 1 diabetes and are already taking insulin, you will find that your insulin needs change as your pregnancy advances. You may need additional injections and blood glucose checks to keep your diabetes controlled.

If you have type 2 diabetes and were able to control blood glucose levels before you were pregnant with meal plans, exercise, and oral medications alone, you will likely need to switch to insulin during pregnancy. Some experts feel that certain diabetes pills are safe to use in pregnancy, while others feel that more research into their use in pregnancy needs to be done. Because the insulin resistance of pregnancy may make pills ineffective, your doctor will probably have you switch to insulin before or when you get pregnant.

It is normal to feel apprehensive about giving yourself a shot. However, with proper technique and with the added convenience of insulin pens and today's very fine needles, insulin injections can be nearly painless and easier than ever to perform.

Types of Insulin

Each type of insulin has a different action time—or the time between when it starts working and how long its effects last. The different action times of insulin are: onset, peak time, and duration. Onset describes the length of time it takes for insulin to reach the blood and begin lowering blood glucose levels; peak describes the time in which insulin is working at its maximum strength; and duration describes the length of time that insulin continues to lower blood glucose levels. The onset, peak, and duration times for the insulins used more commonly during pregnancy are in the table below.

Insulin dosing works by mimicking how insulin works naturally in your body. In people without diabetes, the insulin-producing cells in the pancreas make and release small amounts of insulin throughout the day and night—called basal insulin. The pancreas also releases a short burst of insulin when a person without diabetes eats—this is called bolus insulin. Long-acting insulin works like basal insulin, while rapid-acting and regular insulin are bolus insulin. Intermediate-acting insulin may provide both basal and some bolus effect. Most pregnant women with diabetes take both basal and bolus insulin.

RAPID-ACTING INSULIN

Rapid-acting insulin, also referred to as short-acting insulin, goes to work almost as fast as naturally produced insulin, so it's easy to use when timing insulin with food. It starts to work about 15 minutes after injection. It peaks 1–2 hours after injection, may last up to about 3–5 hours after injection, and is taken right before meals. This insulin works best to handle high blood glucose immediately after eating. The three types of rapid-acting insulin are lispro (Humalog), aspart (Novolog), and glulisine (Apidra).

REGULAR INSULIN

Regular insulin is short acting and is also taken before meals, typically about half an hour before eating. It starts to work 30–60 minutes after injection, peaks 2–3 hours after injection, and lasts for 3–6 hours. Regular insulin is sold under the names of Humulin, Novolin, or ReliOn.

Insulin Commonly Used During Pregnancy

Type of Insulin	Onset	Peak	Duration
RAPID–ACTING			
Humalog (lispro) Novolog (aspart) Apidra (glulisine)	10–15 minutes	30–90 minutes	3–5 hours
SHORT–ACTING			
Regular Humulin Novolin ReliOn	30 minutes– 1 hour	2–3 hours	3–6 hours
INTERMEDIATE			
NPH (N) Humulin N Novolin N ReliOn N	2–4 hours	4–10 hours	10–16 hours
LONG–ACTING			
Lantus (glargine) Levemir (detemir)	2–4 hours	No peak	Up to 24 hours

INTERMEDIATE-ACTING INSULIN

Intermediate-acting insulin (NPH) works more slowly and usually lasts 10–16 hours. It starts to work 2–4 hours after injection and peaks about 4–10 hours after injection. It is also cloudy, rather than clear like other insulin, because it contains suspended crystals that cause it to be absorbed more slowly.

LONG-ACTING INSULIN

Long-acting insulin works for about 24 hours after injected, and does not peak. These insulins start working in 2–4 hours and can stay in the body for 24 hours with little or no peak. Long-acting insulin is injected once or twice a day. This type of insulin is often called "basal" insulin because it is replacing what the body needs between meals and through the night. Levimir and Lantus are the two types of long-acting insulin.

Injecting Insulin

Insulin can be injected at four locations on your body: abdomen (anywhere except within 2 inches of your navel), upper arms (back part), buttocks (anywhere), or thighs (front and outside parts, not inner thighs or right above your knee). Insulin is absorbed at different speeds depending on the area you inject. Your abdomen absorbs insulin the fastest and the most consistently, followed by the arms, buttocks, and thighs.

The abdomen is the preferred site for injection of insulin during pregnancy because it is absorbed the fastest at this site. Using this site will not harm your baby, and because the needle is so short, it will not even reach the muscles of your abdominal wall, much less the uterus.

Rotating the injection sites is another important part of insulin injection. Rotating injection and pump sites is important so that puffy, lumpy spots do not develop and hinder the absorption of insulin. When insulin is injected in the same area over time, it may attract fat into the injection area, leading to the formation of lumps made of fat and scar tissue. Absorption of insulin from these areas is poor. Injecting into these lumps will delay absorption of insulin and blood glucose levels will be difficult to manage. It is important to move the site of insulin injections from one side of your abdomen to the other or to stay at least an inch away from the previous injection. Talk to your health care provider about the best way to rotate insulin injection sites.

How To Make Insulin Injection More Comfortable

▶ Inject insulin at room temperature (once you start using a vial or pen, it does not need to be refrigerated)

▶ Make sure there are no air bubbles in the syringe before you inject

▶ Relax your muscles in the area

▶ Puncture the skin quickly

▶ Keep the needle going in the same direction when you put it in and take it out

▶ Use a new needle each time you inject

PREPARING AND INJECTING INSULIN

Your health care provider will explain how to give insulin injections before you have to do it yourself. Whether it's your first time or you've been doing it for years, it's a good idea to review the basics. It often helps to go over your injection technique with your health care team. Trying to relax before injections can help ease the discomfort because tense muscles can make injections hurt.

Preparing the injection
1. Wash your hands.
2. Choose your injection site.
3. Check the bottle to make sure you are using the right kind of insulin.
4. (For an insulin pen, screw on the needle. Use a new sterile needle every time with insulin pens.)
5. For cloudy insulin, gently roll the bottle of insulin between your palms or rotate the pen slowly from end to end to mix. Make sure it is mixed thoroughly. Shaking the bottle can cause air bubbles. Do not use if it has clumps or particles in it.
6. For a syringe, hold the syringe with the needle pointing up and

draw air into it by pulling down on the plunger to the amount that matches the dose to be given.

7. (For an insulin pen, perform an "air shot" by pushing 1–2 drops of insulin through the needle. Set the insulin dose according to manufacturer's directions. Proceed to instructions for giving the injection, below.)

8. Clean the stopper of the insulin vial with an alcohol swab.

9. Remove the cap from the needle. Draw air into the syringe up to the number of units for your insulin dose. Hold the insulin bottle steady on the tabletop and push the needle straight down into the rubber top on the bottle. Push down on the plunger to inject the air into the insulin bottle.

10. Keep the needle in and turn the bottle and syringe upside down so that the insulin is on top. Pull the correct amount of insulin into the syringe by slowly pulling back on the plunger.

11. Check for air bubbles inside the syringe. If you see air bubbles, keep the bottle upside down and push the plunger up so the insulin goes back into the bottle.

12. Pull down the plunger to refill the syringe. If necessary, empty and refill until all air bubbles in the syringe are gone.

13. Remove the needle from the bottle after checking again that you have the correct dose.

14. If you need to set the syringe down before giving your injection, recap the needle, and lay it on its side. Make sure the needle doesn't touch anything.

Giving the Injection

1. Make sure the site and your hands are clean and dry.

2. Gently pinch a fold of skin between your thumb and forefinger, and inject straight in if you have a normal amount of fatty tissue.

3. Push the needle through the skin as quickly as you can.

4. Relax the pinch and push the plunger in to inject the insulin.

5. Pull the needle straight out. (Don't worry if a drop of blood follows withdrawal of the needle.)

6. Cover the injection site with your finger, a cotton ball, or gauze and apply slight pressure for 5–8 seconds. Do not rub. Rubbing may spread the insulin too quickly or irritate your skin.

7. Write down how much insulin you injected and the time of day.

Talk to your health care providers if you are having problems with any aspect of insulin injection. Be sure to let them know if giving yourself injections is causing a great deal of stress or anxiety, as well. There are several products available that can make injections easier; for example, insertion aids, insulin infusers, and jet injectors. Talk to your health care providers about the different injection tools and how they can make insulin injection easier on you.

STORING INSULIN

Vials of insulin not in use should be stored in the refrigerator. Insulin that is in use can be stored at room temperature to limit local irritation at the injection site. Insulin in vials can be safely stored at room temperature for up to 1 month, while it can be safely stored in the refrigerator until its expiration date. For pens, the length of time they can be used after the first dose depends on the type of insulin. Check the package insert or ask your pharmacist or diabetes educator. However, extreme temperatures (less than 36° or greater than 86°F) should be avoided. After the bottle has been in use for 4 weeks (1 month), loss of potency may occur and that bottle should be replaced.

Check the expiration date before opening your insulin. If the date has passed, don't use the insulin. Any change in color of the insulin, clumping, or precipitation may also mean a loss of potency and that bottle should be replaced.

INSULIN DISPOSAL

An important part of insulin therapy is knowing how to dispose of your syringes, pen needles, and lancets in a safe and proper manner. Syringes, lancets, and any other medical waste that touches human blood is considered medical waste, and must be handled carefully. Check with your care team or local health department to find out if there are rules or special laws for getting rid of medical waste.

Never toss a used syringe directly in a trash can. Place the needle or entire syringe in an opaque (not clear) heavy-duty plastic bottle, like a bleach or detergent bottle with a screw cap or a plastic or medical box that closes firmly. Do not use a container that will allow the needle to break through (e.g., a plastic milk container). When traveling, take your used syringes home. Pack them in a heavy-duty puncture-proof holder for safe transport.

Insulin Pens

The insulin pen is an invention that has revolutionized the convenience and comfort of insulin injections. Insulin pens are popular because they deliver accurate doses and are very convenient. An insulin pen looks just like an ink pen. Instead of a writing tip, it has a disposable needle, and instead of an ink cartridge, there is an insulin cartridge.

You will need to use a new needle every time you inject yourself with an insulin pen. You can buy prefilled disposable pens that you throw away once the insulin cartridge is empty. A variety of insulins are available in pens. You decide the number of units you want, set the injector for that dose, stick the needle in your skin, and inject. It's just that easy. No filling syringes, carrying around syringes, or mixing insulin.

Insulin Pumps

An insulin pump is a battery-powered, computerized device about the size of a cell phone and is attached to the body by a small catheter (plastic tube) inserted beneath the skin into the fat layer. It carries a reservoir of insulin. It can deliver a pre-set amount of insulin continuously, and allows the pump wearer to program the pump to give extra insulin when eating food, which allows more flexibility in when and how you eat. Insulin pumps can also be very helpful for women who have frequent hypoglycemic episodes, frequent fluctuations of their glucose levels, problems with nausea and vomiting, and hypoglycemic symptoms that are not apparent until the glucose levels are dangerously low.

You program the pump to release insulin when you want it to. You tell the pump to give you tiny amounts of insulin continuously throughout the day and night (basal), just the way a normal pancreas would. Then, before each meal, you tell the pump to give you extra insulin just before you eat (bolus). It's important to remember that pumps don't sense your body's need for insulin. They don't adjust by themselves. You still need to monitor your blood glucose levels throughout the day. The pump is worn all the time but can be removed for bathing, swimming, or contact sports. It should not be disconnected for more than an hour at a time. If you are injecting insulin multiple times a day, you may want to consider an insulin pump.

Insulin pumps are convenient because you don't have to stop your daily activities to fill a syringe or prepare an insulin pen. Your insulin is delivered at the push of a button. Pumps are also convenient because they are very precise and can be set to release as little as 1/10 of a unit of insulin per hour. Using an insulin pump is a form of intensive diabetes management, where the aim is to keep blood glucose levels in your target range as much as possible. While the pump adds flexibility and stability to managing your blood glucose levels, it takes time, attention, and energy to learn to use the pump and continue proper use. Talk to your health care provider about whether or not an insulin pump is a good form of diabetes management for you. If so, it's best to start using a pump before you get pregnant so that your blood glucose levels are under control during the first few weeks of pregnancy.

Insulin Needs After Your Baby Is Born

Most women with gestational diabetes will not need any medication after their pregnancies are over, but the woman who has gestational diabetes should have follow-up blood testing within 6 weeks following delivery to be sure of this.

Women who have type 1 diabetes may go through a period of few days immediately following delivery when their insulin requirements decrease dramatically, followed by a gradual return to pre-pregnancy needs. When that happens, it is very important that the new mother monitors her blood glucose frequently and works with her diabetes team to adjust her insulin dose over the next few weeks, until her daily insulin requirements are more stable.

Women who have type 2 diabetes who took pills to lower their blood glucose before they got pregnant, even if they took insulin during pregnancy, may be able to maintain control of their blood glucose with a combination of diet, exercise, and the medication they were taking before they got pregnant. These women also should work with their diabetes team during the post-partum period to determine the best medication regimen. Some oral medications are not recommended if you are breast-feeding.

Oral Medications

Only a small number of studies have been published analyzing the safety and effectiveness of oral medications during pregnancy. Unlike insulin, oral medications cross the placenta to the unborn baby in varying degrees. For both these reasons, the ADA does not recommend their use in pregnancy. However, oral medications are now used more frequently than in the past by some health care providers to manage blood glucose levels that are not controlled by diet and exercise alone during pregnancy. Oral medications are sometimes used as an alternative to insulin, or in some cases, in combination with insulin during pregnancy. The risk and benefits of these medications should be discussed with your health care provider. Two of the oral medications that have been studied for use during pregnancy are glyburide and metformin.

Glyburide works by "pushing" the insulin-producing cells to make more insulin. Several studies have shown that glyburide during pregnancy provides glucose control equivalent to that of insulin in some women who have gestational diabetes. In pregnant women who have a fasting blood glucose over 115 mg/dl, glyburide may not be effective in controlling the blood glucose, making insulin a better choice.

Metformin lowers blood glucose levels by blocking the production of glucose by the liver and by helping muscle and fat to take sugar out of the blood and put it into those cells. It also increases the ability of the body to use the insulin it produces. Some doctors also use metformin to assist women with polycystic ovary disease to become pregnant. Use of the drug in early pregnancy to decrease the risk of miscarriage is controversial. While metformin has not been shown to cause or contribute to birth defects, the appropriate studies to determine this have not been done, and, for ethical reasons, will probably never be done. Finally, many women who are using metformin alone to control their blood glucose levels while pregnant may require insulin in addition to achieve good glucose control.

Neither insulin nor the medications taken by mouth to lower a pregnant woman's blood glucose have been shown to cause harm to an unborn baby. Indeed it is a mother's high blood glucose levels—not her medication—that causes most of the problems to babies of women who have diabetes.

Your meal plan and exercise also affect your insulin regimen. Learn more about how meal planning and exercise play a role in your diabetes management in the next chapter.

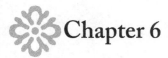Chapter 6

Eating and Exercising for Two

Pregnancy is a great time to change for the better. When you are planning a pregnancy or when you have become pregnant, you often begin to think seriously about your health habits. This is good because what you eat before and during your pregnancy will affect the health of your child. It is also a good time to think about your health for the future. Continuing to eat better and to get regular exercise will help you live a healthier life that will ultimately benefit the health of your children and your family.

Women who have diabetes before becoming pregnant as well as those who are found to have diabetes during pregnancy (gestational diabetes) have some additional dietary and exercise requirements. Although the information in this chapter focuses on healthy eating and exercise habits for pregnancy, the information can be applied to living a healthy lifestyle at any time in your life.

Eating Well During Pregnancy

For most women, the focus of a good meal plan during pregnancy is improving the quality of foods you eat rather than merely increasing the amount of food eaten. A good meal plan is designed to help you avoid high and low blood glucose levels while providing the nutrients your baby needs to grow. When you are pregnant, your body is more insulin resistant, especially in the morning, so you can expect to make changes to what you eat throughout your pregnancy as your baby grows. Many women need to eat less carbohydrate in the morning to manage their blood glucose levels. It is best to avoid drinking juice in the morning.

There is no one perfect food, so including a variety of different foods and watching portion sizes is key to a healthy diet. Also, make sure your choices from each food group provide the highest-quality nutrients you can find. In other words, pick foods rich in vitamins, minerals, and fiber over those that are processed.

General Healthy Eating Tips

Healthy eating is important before, during, and after pregnancy, as well as throughout your life. Healthy eating includes eating a wide variety of foods, including:

- ▶ vegetables
- ▶ whole grains
- ▶ nonfat dairy products
- ▶ fruits
- ▶ beans
- ▶ lean meats
- ▶ poultry
- ▶ fish

Many people think that eating for two means eat a lot more than you did before. This isn't true. You only need to increase your calorie intake by about 300 more calories each day. This is equal to a glass of low-fat milk, a piece of fruit, and a slice of whole-grain bread. Hunger is the easiest way to judge if you are consuming enough calories from day to day. In the long term, monitor your weight gain. Three meals and three snacks a day are common. It may be beneficial to meet with your dietitian during each trimester of your pregnancy to update the plan based on the changing needs of your body and your baby.

Protein needs also increase during pregnancy to support your baby's development. Total needs average about 70 grams of protein per day, or 25 grams more than before pregnancy. Most adults get at least 70 grams of protein daily, but if this is not the case your dietitian can advise you about the types of foods to add. Foods high in protein include dairy products, meat, chicken, fish, eggs, nuts, seeds, and legumes, such as black beans.

If you are trying to eat a consistent amount of carbohydrate, you may want to try the plate method for meal planning. The plate method was designed to help you assemble healthy meals in the correct proportions and to spread the carbohydrate content of the meal evenly within each meal. Focus on filling your plate with nonstarchy vegetables and having smaller portions of starchy foods and meats. Plus, the plate method is a simple way to get started managing your blood glucose levels.

Start by drawing an imaginary line down the center of your plate. On one side, cut it again so you should have three sections on your plate. Fill the largest section with nonstarchy vegetables, such as spinach, carrots, cabbage, green beans, or broccoli. In one of the small sections, include starchy foods, such as whole-grain breads, rice, pasta, beans, or peas. In the other small section, put your meat or meat substitutes, such as chicken, turkey, fish, shrimp, beef, or pork. Add an 8-ounce glass of nonfat or low-fat milk and a piece of fruit to round out your meal. Your plate will look a little different at breakfast. Use half of your plate for starchy foods. You can add fruit in the small part and a meat or meat substitute in the other.

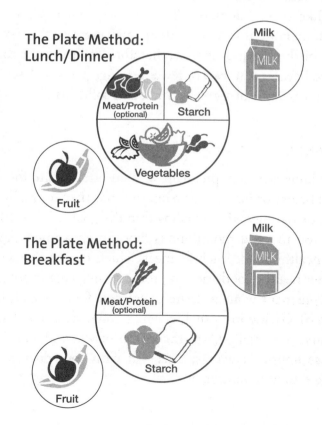

The Plate Method: Lunch/Dinner

Milk · MILK

Meat/Protein (optional) · Starch

Fruit

Vegetables

The Plate Method: Breakfast

Milk · MILK

Meat/Protein (optional)

Fruit

Starch

HEALTHY BEVERAGES

Staying hydrated during pregnancy will help deliver nutrients to your baby and reduce constipation and fatigue. Drinking water is also important if you are vomiting or have diarrhea. Drink at least 8 cups (8 ounces each) of water daily and supplement it with beverages that add nutrients, not just sugar. Skim milk is a good choice as well as fruit or smoothies. Avoid beverages providing empty calories such as sodas, sweetened fruit drinks, punches, and sweetened, high-fat coffee beverages or milk shakes. The US FDA has determined that artificial sweeteners are safe for people with diabetes and during pregnancy. If you have any questions about whether it is safe to use them during pregnancy, you can talk to your health care provider.

Alcoholic beverages are known to harm the development of your baby. Because it is not worth the pleasure of a few drinks to risk causing *any* harm to your baby, you are advised to not drink at all during pregnancy. It is also wise to keep caffeine to a minimum by limiting caffeinated coffees, teas, and diet sodas. Caffeine has not been shown to cause direct damage to the baby like alcohol does, but there is disagreement about a safe level of consumption. High intakes of caffeine may increase the risk of miscarriage or low birth weight. It is wise, therefore, to limit your consumption of caffeinated beverages to two or fewer servings per day. A serving means a small (6 ounce) cup, not a *grande* drink at a coffee bar.

FOOD CRAVINGS

For some unknown reason, pregnant women often desire foods they had never craved before or have an aversion to foods they normally like. These cravings can be harmless if they fall within the goals of a healthy diet and don't cause you to eat a monotonous diet. Some women experience an aversion to healthy foods, such as meat, which can be managed by substituting other healthy foods rich in protein (milk, yogurt, tofu, beans). In a few cases, pregnant women desire to eat non-food items (dirt, clay, ice, laundry starch). Giving in to such cravings could replace nutritious foods in the diet and potentially harm the health of you and your baby. If you develop these unusual cravings, discuss it with your doctor. Sometimes they are linked to iron deficiency.

MORNING SICKNESS

"Morning sickness" (nausea and vomiting) is a misnomer because it can occur at any time during the day, although many women find it worse when the stomach is empty. It is usually most severe in the first trimester and fades thereafter. If you are taking insulin to lower your blood glucose and you cannot hold down foods or liquids, call your doctor immediately, since there is a danger of low blood glucose. Your doctor might prescribe anti-nausea medication or even admit you to the hospital if your vomiting can't be controlled.

Morning sickness occurs in many pregnancies in the first trimester. Pregnancies complicated by diabetes are no different. If you are experiencing significant morning sickness, your doctor may want to prescribe a medication for it. If you had diabetes before you were pregnant and are taking insulin or another medication that lowers your blood glucose, nausea and vomiting may affect your appetite and your sugar levels. You and your doctor may need to work on adjusting your insulin dose in response to this.

Tips To Help Avoid Nausea

The following simple practices may help reduce mild nausea.

▶ Avoid eating too much at any one time.

▶ Eat slowly and don't skip meals.

▶ Avoid strong food odors that bother you.

▶ Drink plenty of fluids, especially if you are vomiting (try drinking frequent small sips). Carbonated beverages are often easier to keep down.

▶ Make sure you get enough sleep and rest.

CONSTIPATION

Constipation is common during pregnancy. One reason is that your intestinal muscles become more relaxed. Another reason is that, as your baby grows, there is more pressure on your intestines. If you have problems with constipation, try the following:

▶ Drink plenty of liquids, especially water.

▶ Eat high-fiber foods, including whole grains, bran cereal, and vegetables.

▶ Get regular exercise.

If the problem persists, discuss it with your health care providers.

HEARTBURN

As your pregnancy progresses, you may get heartburn. Some of the symptoms of heartburn include burning discomfort in the stomach or throat, an upset stomach, or a stomachache. The following may help:

▶ Eat frequent, small meals that include protein.

▶ Eat more foods with calcium and magnesium in them.

▶ Avoid acidic or spicy foods.

▶ Eat slowly; be sure to chew food well.

▶ Avoid eating right before bedtime.

If heartburn persists, check with your health care provider for help.

Insulin and Your Meal Plan

If your doctor determines that you need to take insulin during your pregnancy to control your blood glucose, it is very important to eat according to the schedule you will make with your doctor and/or dietitian. Pregnant women are usually prescribed a combination of long-acting (NPH) and short- or rapid-acting insulin. The long-acting insulin lasts all day, and the short acting works over a few hours after a meal.

When you take insulin, it is very important to eat on a schedule or you run the risk of low blood glucose, which is dangerous to your health and that of your baby. Skipping meals or eating at odd hours can cause your blood glucose to be too low or too high. The best way to maintain blood glucose levels is to learn how carbohydrates affect your blood glucose levels and learn to determine how much insulin you need to use depending on the foods you are eating.

Carbohydrates are often the most talked-about source of calories when it comes to diabetes—this is because they're your body's main source of energy, and because they are directly linked to the rise in blood glucose after meals.. After you eat, your body breaks down carbohydrates into glucose that travels to the bloodstream. Examples of foods containing carbohydrates are: bread, cereal, pasta, starchy vegetables (peas, corn, and potatoes) soda, ice cream, fruit, and dairy products like yogurt and milk. If you are using insulin, a dietitian can help you match the amount of carbohydrate eaten to the amount of insulin you will need to keep blood glucose levels from rising. Women who had diabetes before pregnancy will often count carbohydrates and learn the "insulin to carbohydrate" ratio that works for them. Women with gestational diabetes usually learn to eat consistent amounts of carbohydrate at each meal, and will sometimes be told to restrict the amount or types of carbohydrate in their diet.

Your doctor and/or dietitian should teach you all of the details of diet planning on insulin. Make sure you call them or schedule extra visits if you are confused about your diet or medication. Learning to use insulin (see chapter 5) is a skill that can take some time, so don't be shy about asking for help.

Dietary Supplements

Eating a balanced diet before and during pregnancy is important for many reasons, but there are a few critical nutrients—iron, folic acid, and calcium—that are difficult to get from diet alone for the needs of pregnancy. Most physicians recommend taking a prenatal vitamin/mineral supplement to ensure that nutrient deficiencies do not occur. Most products labeled "prenatal vitamins" contain iron, folic acid, and calcium in quantities adequate to make up the additional requirements for pregnancy. It is important to remember that supplements do not replace healthy eating; they *supplement* it. This is because the foods we eat contain many other nutrients besides vitamins and minerals that are also important for our health.

Recently, there has been a lot of interest in fish oil supplements for pregnant women. Fish oil contains high levels of omega-3 fatty acids, especially DHA (docosahexaenoic acid). Higher intakes of DHA from fish or fish oils may help prevent preterm birth, but it is uncertain if there are benefits for women having normal pregnancies. Unfortunately, some fish also contain mercury and other environmental toxins and pesticides, and national guidelines suggest that pregnant women avoid mercury-containing foods. Talk to your care team about what amounts of fish are advisable. Other food sources of omega-3 fatty acids include walnuts, flaxseeds, canola oil, and omega-3 enriched eggs.

Herbal supplements have recently been promoted in books, magazines, and websites as remedies for the discomforts of pregnancy. The ingestion, however, of herbal medicines that contain large amounts of biologically active compounds is risky for pregnant women. For example, ginger, garlic, ginkgo, and ginseng all have been reported to adversely affect blood circulation and could increase bleeding during labor. Be wary of herbal supplements that have not been tested for safety and limit the herbs you use to those added during food preparation or in conventional herbal teas.

Weight Matters

Most women need to gain some weight during pregnancy. Even if a woman is overweight when she gets pregnant, she will gain some weight from the weight of the baby and extra body tissues and fluids.

The amount of weight gain recommended during pregnancy is different for women of different pre-pregnancy BMIs. The higher the BMI, the *less* weight you need to gain during pregnancy. While pregnancy is not a time to lose weight, it is a great time to make healthy changes to your diet and exercise habits, as mentioned earlier. If you do this, you can actually be healthier after your baby is born than you were before you got pregnant.

Women who are overweight or obese prior to pregnancy have higher risks of some pregnancy complications, including gestational diabetes and type 2 diabetes. Heavier women also have higher risks of having larger and heavier babies. These larger babies may make childbirth more difficult and increase the chances of needing a cesarean delivery. Larger babies also may have some medical complications in the first few weeks after birth, and they may also be more likely to be overweight later in life and develop diabetes and other diseases.

Women who are overweight or obese at the time they get pregnant can reduce these risks if they don't gain more weight than is recommended by the guidelines. You and your prenatal care provider should set a goal together for your weight gain during pregnancy. At each prenatal visit you should discuss how much weight has been gained. If you find that you are gaining weight more quickly than expected, you are not alone—many women gain more than the recommended amount and it can be difficult to prevent excess weight gain. However, there may be steps you can take to slow the gain down. Your prenatal care provider and a dietitian can help you to do this in a healthy way. Rather than focusing on the total weight you gain, it is more important to consider your pattern of weight gain. If you start to gain a lot of weight suddenly or if you stop gaining weight or even start losing weight, you should talk to your health care team right away to determine the reason.

Common Weight Goals for Pregnancy

If your pre-pregnancy weight is...   *Then gain...*

If your pre-pregnancy weight is...	Then gain...
Underweight (BMI less than 18.5 kg/m²)	28–40 pounds
Normal (BMI 18.5–24.9 kg/m²)	25–35 pounds
Overweight (BMI 25–29.9 kg/m²)	15–25 pounds
Obese (BMI 30 kg/m² or higher)	11–20 pounds

These are averages to give you an idea of how much weight you should gain. Talk to your health care provider about your specific weight goals during pregnancy. (Adapted from *ADA Complete Guide to Diabetes*, 5th Edition, ADA, 2011).

High weight gain *early* in pregnancy increases the risk of getting gestational diabetes. If you have already been diagnosed with diabetes, you can still have a healthier pregnancy if you can keep weight gain in check through good diet and exercise habits. Women with gestational diabetes who gain too much weight are more likely to need insulin to keep their blood glucose in control. Women who have any type of diabetes may have babies who, despite being of normal weight, may have a greater proportion of their birth weight as fat weight. These babies' excess fat may increase the likelihood of their developing high blood pressure, obesity, diabetes, and heart disease as children, adolescents, and adults. There is now evidence that women who have gestational diabetes may decrease both the baby's birth weight and the proportion of birth weight that is fat by lowering their blood glucose levels and limiting their weight gain during pregnancy.

Some women do not gain very much weight during pregnancy. If you are eating a healthy diet with three meals a day and two snacks, and you are eating the recommended amounts of protein, fats, and carbohydrates, and you still gain less weight than recommended, you don't need to worry. You will want to discuss your diet in detail with your provider and/or dietitian to make sure it is adequate in nutrients, however. Your provider may want to check the growth of the baby with ultrasound, but in most cases, the baby grows just fine. If you were overweight or obese at the time you got pregnant and you don't gain much weight in spite of a healthy diet, you actually have a lower risk of pregnancy complications compared to women who gain more weight.

Teenagers who become pregnant may need to eat more calories than most other women. Because the body of a teenager is still growing, the teen mother needs to provide for her own body's growth as well as for her baby's. Your health care provider can help you determine a goal weight.

What To Do if Weight Gain Is Too Fast/Too High?

▶ Increase your physical activity—walk after meals, swim, ride a stationary bike

▶ Meet with a dietitian to discuss your diet

▶ Increase the amount of fiber in your diet, especially from fresh vegetables

▶ Reduce or eliminate "junk food" like cakes, cookies, candy, chips, and other foods that are high in calories.

▶ Eliminate juice, soda, and other sweetened drinks—replace with water, fat-free milk, or decaffeinated tea

▶ Make sure you are getting enough sleep

▶ Take steps to reduce stress (meditation, yoga, spending time outdoors, seek out support of friends and family)

Staying Active During Pregnancy

Pregnant women frequently question whether it is safe to exercise during pregnancy. Regular physical activity is not only safe for pregnant women, it benefits health by offsetting some of the problems of pregnancy, such as varicose veins, leg cramps, fatigue, and constipation. It can also help maintain the muscle tone of the abdomen, uterus, and vagina, and can help prevent urinary incontinence and lower back pain. Pregnant women are more susceptible to metabolic disorders like high blood pressure, high blood glucose, and diabetes. Regular physical activity can help alleviate these problems. For women who have diabetes, exercise, especially following meals, may help the muscles use the glucose in the bloodstream, and help keep blood glucose in good control. It is usually safe to continue any exercises you were doing before you became pregnant, or begin a moderate exercise such as walking; however, pregnancy is not the time to take up new, strenuous levels of activity. Talk to your health care team about the exercise plan that is right for you.

Tips to Exercising Safely During Pregnancy

▶ Start your workout with at least a 5-minute warm-up and 5 minutes of stretching. This will help your muscles get loose.

▶ Wear loose-fitting, comfortable clothes.

▶ Wear comfortable, supportive athletic shoes.

▶ Exercise on a flat, level surface.

▶ Drink water before, during, and after you exercise.

▶ Test your blood glucose before and after exercise to make sure it hasn't gone too low.

▶ Cool down with 5 minutes of light walking and 5 minutes of stretching.

A good physical activity program during pregnancy includes cardiovascular exercise, muscle strengthening, muscle endurance, and flexibility. Good, safe cardiovascular exercises include walking, swimming, water aerobics, stationary bikes or low-impact cardiovascular machines, and low-impact aerobics. It is always wise to stretch your arms, legs, back, neck, and shoulder area before and after a workout to prevent muscle stiffness and promote flexibility.

As pregnancy advances, your body will become structurally stressed as the weight of the baby pulls on your spine and forces your lower back to hollow and your abdominal muscles to lengthen. Specific exercises to strengthen the core muscles of the abdomen, lower back, and pelvic floor can prevent some of the discomfort from your baby's stress on the spine and lower back. Several websites, such as http://www.webmd.com/baby/guide/pregnancy-safe-exercises, provide a simple series of stretches you can do during pregnancy. You can also ask your health care team to advise you. Remember: consult your health care team before you start any exercise regimen. Your health care team will give you personal exercise guidelines, based on your medical history.

Activities To Avoid During Pregnancy

Although appropriate exercises are an integral part of a healthy pregnancy, you should avoid any activities that could cause injury to your baby. Activities to avoid include the following.

▶ Activities that put you in danger of falling or receiving abdominal injury, such as contact sports (basketball or soccer) or fast-paced outdoor sports (skiing)

▶ Activities putting pressure on your abdomen, such as exercises done lying on your stomach

▶ Scuba diving

▶ Vigorous, intense exercise, such as running too fast to carry on a conversation

▶ Activities with bouncing or jolting movements (horseback riding or high-impact aerobics)

In general, pregnant women need to avoid putting stress on their abdominal area or lower back, avoid exercise with a risk of injury or discomfort, and avoid activities that do not accommodate to the changes of posture and balance that come with pregnancy.

Having diabetes requires some special attention during exercise. Because exercising accelerates the rate at which your muscles use glucose for energy, you may experience low blood glucoses (hypoglycemia) while or after exercising. It is important that you test your blood glucose before and after exercise, recognize the signs of hypoglycemia, stop exercising if you experience these symptoms and check your blood glucose, and know how to treat hypoglycemia (see chapter 4).

Chapter 7

Labor and Delivery

The big day is here! After nine months of being pregnant, you will finally get to meet your new baby. You have been looking forward to this day for a long time. During the last few weeks of your pregnancy, your health care providers have studied your health and that of your growing baby and discussed with you the best time and method for delivery. You can expect to have a safe and successful delivery while your care providers take the necessary steps to assure the health of you and your baby throughout delivery.

To help you prepare for labor, many hospitals and other organizations offer classes (such as Lamaze) to help you have a smooth delivery. They teach you what to expect during delivery, techniques to improve delivery and to relieve pain during labor, and how to care for your baby after birth. Because of the care needed for both mom and baby during and after delivery, home births are not advised for women with diabetes. You can ask your health care provider or check with your hospital about prepared childbirth classes in your area.

It's also important to have a partner or coach helping your throughout the labor and delivery process. This can be a spouse, parent, relative, or friend. Having a support system with you before and during the birth can help you be more relaxed during your time at the hospital.

This chapter was designed to let you know what special care you may receive during your birth experience because you have diabetes. Please bear in mind that your delivery experience will probably be very similar to that of a woman who does not have diabetes.

Don't be alarmed if there are quite a few people in the room during the delivery. Besides the doctor, there may be a nurse or two, possibly an anesthesiologist, a resident doctor or students if you are at a teaching hospital, and very often a pediatrician. This does not mean there is anything wrong, but many hospitals want a pediatrician present at the delivery just to be on the safe side, to make sure the baby can receive immediate assistance, if needed.

Timing of Delivery

There are several factors that your doctor needs to consider before deciding when would be the best time to deliver your baby. Your own health, the estimated size of the baby, how well your blood glucose is controlled, the results of your sonogram and of antepartum testing—all these need to be taken into account.

To determine the safest time and method to deliver your baby, your health care team will examine a variety of factors: blood glucose control, blood pressure, kidney function, and any diabetes complications you may have. The team will also study your baby's size and movements, his or her heart-rate pattern, and the amount of amniotic fluid in the uterus.

In some cases, a small amount of fluid will be withdrawn from your uterus—known as amniocentesis. This procedure will help determine whether your baby's lungs are mature and help guide the timing of delivery. Your provider may suggest that you get an injection of betamethasone, a steroid that will help increase your baby's lung maturity, if it looks like your baby will be delivered early. While you are in labor, your baby's heart rate will be tracked by a fetal monitor.

If you have gestational diabetes that is well controlled and the baby is not too big, your doctor will most likely wait for you to go into labor on your own. This is called "spontaneous labor."

If you have type 1 or type 2 diabetes and your blood glucose levels are not within your target range or you have frequent bouts of hyperglycemia, or if the baby appears to be growing too big, your doctor may decide to make you go into labor, if you haven't gone into labor on your own. This is called "induction of labor," and usually means that you will be getting a medication called Pitocin (oxytocin) through your vein that will make your uterus contract. Before getting the Pitocin, your doctor may decide to give you a medication called prostaglandin to soften and prepare your cervix for labor.

In general, your doctor will decide to induce your labor if he or she thinks that it might not be safe for you or for your baby to continue the pregnancy. In addition, your doctor has to take into account the size of the baby. Women with diabetes tend to have larger babies, especially if the blood glucose was not controlled very well during the pregnancy. It may be more difficult to deliver a large baby that has a lot of fat. There is also a risk that the shoulders will get stuck after the head comes out; this is called "shoulder dystocia," and it is more common in babies of mothers with diabetes.

There are several other situations that might prompt your doctor to induce your labor. For instance, if your blood pressure goes up and you develop a condition called preeclampsia, your doctor may decide to induce your labor. Preeclampsia can be dangerous for the mother and baby if it does not respond to bed rest or medications. This condition is somewhat more common in women who have diabetes. Whatever the cause, your doctor will explain the rationale for induction to you and discuss with you what to expect. Make sure to ask any questions that you might have. Having your questions answered will help you feel more relaxed so you can focus on the birth of your baby.

Cesarean Section

Most pregnant women, including women with diabetes, deliver their babies by a vaginal delivery. However, one in every 3 to 4 women in the general population of the United States delivers by cesarean section (also called C-section). During a C-section, an incision is made through your abdomen and uterus, through which the baby is removed.

There are three main reasons to deliver by C-section: because the baby is showing signs of not doing well during labor and needs to be delivered quickly; because labor is not progressing and the baby simply won't come out; or because the mother has already had a previous C-section and she and her doctor have agreed to schedule a repeat C-section. All these considerations apply to women with diabetes as well. If you are having a large baby, a C-section may be recommended to avoid the risk of shoulder dystocia.

Cesarean deliveries, though relatively safe and frequent, put women at higher risk for infections, increased bleeding, prolonged recovery, and other issues. The surgery itself usually lasts less than an hour, and requires you to stay 3–4 days in the hospital. After surgery, it will take you 4–6 weeks to recover and to gradually get back to normal activity. This is in contrast to the 24- to 36-hour stay that usually follows an uncomplicated vaginal delivery.

Even though C-section is overall a very safe operation, it does have potential risks, just like any other surgical procedure. In women who have diabetes, there is an increased risk of infection and of poor healing of the wound. This is especially true in women who are overweight and women who have pre-existing complications of type 1 or type 2 diabetes. Discuss possible complications with your health care provider and ask any questions you may have about the procedure.

Having a C-section does not necessarily mean that you will have to deliver by C-section in future pregnancies. Most women can try having a vaginal delivery after having a previous C-section.

Testing and Monitoring During Labor

During labor, your baby's heart rate and well-being will probably be monitored by a fetal monitor that is placed on the outside of your abdomen or by an internal monitor that is attached to your baby's head after your water has broken. Not all pregnancies require monitoring of the baby's heart rate throughout labor. But when the mother has diabetes, the disease may affect the baby's ability to tolerate labor.

In the labor room, the nurse initially will place a strap around your abdomen and connect two transducers to the strap. One will register your contractions and the other will register the baby's heart rate. Later in labor, after your water breaks, the external monitoring devices may be replaced by a tube placed through your vagina into your uterus to measure the pressure of your contractions and by a wire attached to your baby's scalp to register the baby's heart rate.

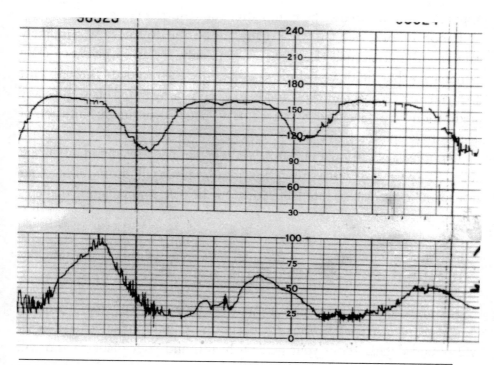

The image above shows what you will see on the monitor during labor. The top panel shows the baby's heart rate, while the bottom panel shows your contractions. (Medical Management of Pregnancy Complicated by Diabetes, ADA, 2009)

Controlling Blood Glucose During Labor

Keeping your blood glucose levels as close to normal as possible will be a major concern during your labor and delivery, regardless of when or how your baby is delivered. Keeping your blood glucose in your target range during labor will decrease the risk that your baby's blood glucose will drop after birth. Labor, like any strenuous exercise, tends to lower blood glucose levels in a person whose diabetes is well controlled, so you will probably need less insulin during active labor. Your blood glucose will be checked frequently (probably every few hours) and your insulin and glucose regimen will be tailored to your needs during this time.

If you have type 1 diabetes and use an insulin pump, bring it with you to the hospital. Women who use a pump regularly and are having a vaginal delivery are often able to keep their pump on during labor and delivery.

You will also want to use the pump after you deliver.

Labor is work, and you will usually not be able to eat, so it is unlikely your blood glucose will rise. You will probably get an intravenous (IV) catheter so that fluids or calories can be given as needed. Through this line, you will receive sufficient fluids to keep you hydrated, as well as any medications you may need. Some women will get a continuous infusion of insulin to keep blood glucose controlled.

If you have gestational diabetes, you may not need insulin at all during labor. At the start of active labor, your insulin needs will drop. Talk to your care team before you go into labor to know the plan for managing diabetes during this time.

Medications During Labor

The contractions of labor can become very painful, and many women choose to receive medications to relieve the pain. Your anesthesiologist will obtain details about your general health and your diabetes and will suggest the best method of pain relief for you.

Most women with diabetes may get regional anesthesia through an epidural catheter. The anesthesiologist will insert a needle through your lower back and thread a thin catheter (a very narrow tube) into the space around your spinal cord. Medications administered through the catheter will help relieve the pain. Usually, you will also feel numbness in your legs, but this will wear off after the delivery.

Sometimes, due to other medical conditions, or due to complications of pre-existing diabetes, the anesthesiologist will not be able to give you epidural anesthesia and will have to find a different method to help you cope with the pain, such as medications administered through your vein.

After your baby arrives, your body begins to recover from the hard work of pregnancy and delivery. Your hard work has paid off and you have a beautiful new baby to care for.

Chapter 8

After-Delivery Care
for Mother and Baby

This chapter focuses on post-delivery care for you and your baby. Your diabetes care will change after delivery, depending on the type of diabetes you had. Your health care team can help you answer any questions you may have concerning after-delivery care for you and your baby.

After you deliver the baby, if you have a vaginal birth, your doctor will make sure your placenta comes out and that you are not bleeding too much, and will repair any tears that might have occurred during delivery. In the meantime, the nurse or the pediatrician will make sure your baby is doing well. You will usually be able to hold your baby right away or very soon after delivery, and enjoy his or her closeness during the first moments of life.

It is very good for your baby to cry because this opens up his or her lungs and helps the baby breath efficiently. This is a new experience for the baby because while being in your womb, you were supplying the baby with all its needs including oxygen and there was no need for it to use its lungs. But as soon as the baby is born, the lungs need to inflate and start delivering oxygen, so it is important for the baby to cry vigorously immediately after birth.

As things are settling down in the delivery room, the nurse will check the baby's blood glucose to make sure it is not dropping. During pregnancy, your blood glucose was transferred to the baby's blood through the placenta. If your blood glucose levels were high during pregnancy, the baby had to produce his or her own insulin in a much higher amount than normal. After delivery, your baby's body continues to make extra insulin, which in turn may lead to low blood glucose levels. If the glucose is low but the baby is otherwise doing well, early feedings will be started. If the baby cannot feed very well, or if glucose is very low before or even after feedings, glucose may be given through an IV and the baby will be monitored in the neonatal intensive care unit (NICU) until his or blood glucose levels stabilize. Most hospitals have a policy to check the baby's blood glucose level at least twice within the first hour after birth.

Your Blood Glucose Levels After Delivery

Your blood glucose levels may remain low for several hours after delivery. If you have type 1 diabetes, your doctor will tell you how to adjust your insulin doses after the delivery. Your body needs much less insulin immediately after the pregnancy is over, usually one-third to one-half of the doses you were on before delivery. Therefore, you have to be careful to not overdose yourself and end up with hypoglycemia (low blood glucose). Blood glucose monitoring is the best way to chart these changes and will make it easier to make the necessary adjustments as your body returns to its non-pregnant state. A few weeks after delivery, your insulin dose should return to the levels you used before you became pregnant. (See more about how your medications will change after delivery in Chapter 9.)

It is best to check your blood glucose very frequently following delivery to avoid either high or low levels until you get an idea of how much insulin your body needs. Your health care providers will check your blood glucose levels while you're resting.

If you have type 2 diabetes, your doctor will decide which medication you should take after the delivery. You will usually be able to go back to the same medications you were taking before pregnancy, as long as they were controlling your diabetes well, although this may have to be modified if you are breastfeeding.

If you have gestational diabetes, there is a very good chance that your diabetes will go away immediately after the delivery. This is especially true if your diabetes was controlled with a meal plan and exercise during pregnancy. Pregnancy changes the way your body responds to your own insulin, but once the pregnancy is over, your body goes back to responding the way it did before pregnancy. You should continue to check your blood glucose levels for at least several days to make sure your diabetes is actually gone.

Some women who had gestational diabetes may continue to have high blood glucose levels even after delivery. This is usually because they had some form of diabetes before pregnancy but simply were not aware of it. This is more likely to happen in women whose diabetes was diagnosed during the first few months of pregnancy.

If you had gestational diabetes, even if your blood glucose normalizes after delivery, your doctor will recommend that you return for a glucose tolerance test 4–6 weeks after delivery to check and see if you still have diabetes (see chapter 9).

Breastfeeding

Breastfeeding has health benefits for both mother and baby. In one study, babies that were breastfed for six months or more, after exposure to their mother's diabetes in the womb, were no more likely to put on extra weight as children (ages 6–13) than those who were not exposed to diabetes. This has shown to decrease risk of type 2 diabetes for the child. Breast-fed babies also develop fewer allergies and stomach complaints and experience fewer early childhood infections. There is some evidence that the risk of type 1 diabetes may also be lowered.

Along with benefits for the baby, breastfeeding may help the mother to get her own glucose under control. It may also help to decrease the risk for a woman with gestational diabetes to develop type 2 diabetes later.

Breastfeeding may also help you lose the weight you gained during pregnancy, although you shouldn't try to lose it too quickly. While you are breastfeeding, it is important that you get the right amounts of fluids, protein, vitamins, and minerals. Most nursing mothers will need about 2,200 calories a day to produce high-quality milk. Working with your dietitian, you should be able to develop a meal plan that will allow you to achieve gradual weight loss and still be successful at breastfeeding.

If you have type 1 or type 2 diabetes and use either insulin or oral blood glucose lowering–medications, it's important to understand the safety of these medications while breastfeeding. Most medications used to treat diabetes can be used safely during breastfeeding. The American Academy of Pediatrics considers most oral medications used to lower blood sugar (glucose) to be safe breastfeeding, even though small amounts of some of these medications do get into breast milk. Check with your doctor to find out if your medications are OK to continue using while breastfeeding. Insulin does not get into breast milk and is considered safe for breastfeeding. You should work with your doctor to determine which medication is best for you during breastfeeding.

Breastfeeding Tips

Breastfeeding is good for women with diabetes, but it may make your blood glucose a little harder to predict. To help prevent low blood glucose levels due to breastfeeding, try these tips:

▶ Plan to have a snack before or during nursing.

▶ Drink enough fluids (plan to sip a glass of water or a caffeine-free drink while nursing).

▶ Keep something to treat low blood glucose nearby when you nurse, so you don't have to stop a feeding to treat low blood glucose levels.

Women who breastfeed use more calories than women who don't breastfeed. What you drink and eat can affect your milk supply, as well as your blood glucose. You may find that breastfeeding will cause your blood glucose level to drop fairly quickly, especially at night. You may need to change your overnight dosage or add a snack with late night feedings. You will need to work with your doctor and dietitian to adjust your meal plan while you are nursing.

Women who have diabetes or gestational diabetes may face some special challenges in establishing breastfeeding. Cesarean birth, birth before 39 weeks, or pre-existing diabetes may mean that your baby will be in a special care (neonatal) unit for some time after birth and this may make it difficult for you to establish breastfeeding in the early days after delivery. Most obstetric units now appreciate the need for skin-to-skin contact between mother and baby, and for breastfeeding. Breastfeeding babies in the neonatal intensive care unit (NICU), as well as breast pumping for very premature babies, have become common practices.

Make sure that you ask your doctor and your baby's pediatrician about breastfeeding support programs and the availability of lactation counselors at the hospital where you plan to deliver. With a little planning and persistence, you should be able to establish breastfeeding before you and your baby are discharged from the hospital.

Although breastfeeding may be an excellent way to nourish your baby, you may be unable or unwilling to breastfeed. Some women are uncomfortable breastfeeding, have jobs that make breastfeeding on a regular schedule difficult, or have other reasons to not breastfeed. It is important that you understand the benefits of breastfeeding to your baby and yourself, as well as the work entailed in breastfeeding. If you are unable or unwilling to breastfeed, don't feel guilty. Your baby can still get the nutrients he or she needs, and the close bonding to you, from bottle-feeding formula.

Your Baby After Delivery

Despite the best of efforts, babies of mothers who have diabetes can run into some problems. Most of these are minor, and do not have any permanent effects on the baby. Your baby's blood glucose will be tested after delivery. Your baby's doctor will explain to you if additional tests are needed, what those tests are for, and what additional treatments your baby might need. Some problems that can occur in the babies born to mothers with diabetes are listed below.

JAUNDICE

Many newborn babies develop *jaundice*—or yellowing of the skin and eyes caused by increased levels of bilirubin. Bilirubin is a waste product of red blood cells that is excreted by the liver. The livers of newborns are not mature enough to get rid of all the bilirubin, and the incompletely formed bilirubin is dispersed to different parts of the body. When it appears in the skin, a yellow color develops.

While many healthy babies develop jaundice, it seems to appear more often in babies of mothers who have diabetes. This may be related to a higher amount of red blood cells being present at birth.

Most of the time, the baby's bilirubin level is not very high and does not need special treatment. If the bilirubin level is higher, the first treatment is to expose the baby's skin to a special light. This is called phototherapy. Depending on the baby's level of jaundice and clinical condition this treatment may be given in the nursery, NICU, or at home. If your baby is still being treated for jaundice after a couple of days, you may have to go home while he or she is still at the hospital.

POLYCYTHEMIA

Sometimes a baby will be born with an excessive amount of red blood cells. Infants of diabetic mothers, especially those of women whose blood glucose levels have run high during pregnancy, are at increased risk of having more red blood cells than normal. This condition is called *polycythemia*. Sometimes babies who have severe polycythemia need a part of their blood replaced with salt water to bring the concentration of red blood cells down. This is done to prevent damage to the baby's kidneys and brain by the excessive number of red cells clogging up the blood vessels in these organs.

LOW CALCIUM AND MAGNESIUM

Sometimes babies are found to have low levels of calcium shortly after birth. Calcium is a mineral in the body that is necessary for a variety of body functions, including building bones and making our heart and muscles work. Most of the time it does not need any treatment unless the baby shows signs of low calcium. If that happens your baby may need extra calcium by mouth or through an IV. Occasionally, a baby may need special formula with increased calcium for few days if he or she is not being breastfed. The baby may also be at higher risk for low magnesium levels, which are often related to calcium levels. A low magnesium level resolves by itself most of the time.

BREATHING PROBLEMS

While breathing problems are rare in babies born after 38 weeks, they are seen more often in babies born before 38 weeks. A common breathing problem is called *respiratory distress syndrome* (RDS). In RDS, the baby's lungs have not developed enough for the baby to be able to breathe on his or her own.

Some (particularly large) babies can develop a condition called *transient tachypnea of the newborn* (TTN). "Tachypnea" means rapid breathing. In this condition, the baby breathes rapidly and needs oxygen for 2–3 days. The tachypnea usually lasts for a short time period.

Babies affected by RDS or TTN most often need care in the NICU where they will receive oxygen, and, on occasion, ventilator support until they are able to breathe on their own.

The above problems are more common in babies whose mothers had diabetes. While it is unusual for your baby to have any of these issues after birth, it is useful to know something about these possible complications so you can be prepared in the event that your baby has to stay in the hospital a few extra days after delivery.

Chapter 9

Balancing Life as a New Mom

Having a new baby in the house is both exciting and stressful. If this is your first baby, it marks the start of a brand-new phase of your life. New mothers often feel overwhelmed by the nature of this commitment and tend to put all their time and effort into being "the best mother" possible.

With your baby's arrival, your focus turns to caring for your little one. Keep in mind that to take good care of your baby you need to take good care of yourself. Stick to your habits that helped you keep your blood glucose levels on target during pregnancy. And remember: It's OK to ask for help. Enlist family and friends to watch the baby or make dinner or straighten up the house. You have just learned a lot about meal planning, exercise, and healthy eating. You have developed routines to achieve these goals and should continue to spend some time each day continuing the good habits. You can help yourself achieve these goals by asking yourself what you want to achieve and what you want to enjoy.

Your Physical and Mental Health

During the first weeks at home with baby, you are likely to be tired, stressed from lack of sleep, and off schedule. Odd sleep patterns increase the danger of napping through a snack or mealtime. Low blood glucose is a real danger. It's important for your baby's safety to avoid blood glucose reactions that could confuse you. For all of the above reasons, it is important to check your blood glucose often during this time. And your records of your blood glucose levels will help you and your team adjust your insulin dose.

While having diabetes doesn't put you at an increased risk for postpartum depression, the extra work of managing your diabetes when you have a newborn (who sleeps only a few hours at a time) can seem near impossible. Postpartum depression can bring sadness, anxiety, mood swings, insomnia, and loss of appetite. More serious signs include thoughts of hurting your baby or yourself. If you suspect you have postpartum depression, talk to your doctor right away. Reaching out to your partner or other family members, too, can help alleviate feelings of being overwhelmed.

Don't forget that diet and exercise are just as important as your medication in controlling your diabetes. It can be very difficult to maintain a focus on your own health once a new baby is brought home. Your efforts to maintain your own treatment schedule may seem less important to you than the needs of your baby and it can be very frustrating to try to balance your needs and those of your baby and your family. Remember—you can function best if you are healthy and not affected by high or low blood glucose levels. Your baby and your family will undergo a lot of changes in the first year, so start with short-term goal setting—a period of a few months.

Tips To Help You Stay Healthy

▶ Watch for signs of depression and talk to your health care provider right away if you think you are experiencing symptoms.

▶ Eat healthy meals and get proper nutrition.

▶ Check your blood glucose levels often.

▶ Sleep whenever you can. Try to rest whenever your baby is sleeping or if he or she (or they, if you have more than one baby) are being cared for by someone else.

▶ Take a few minutes each day just for you: take a warm bath, read, or walk with a friend.

▶ Accept offers of help from friends and family.

▶ Ask for help.

How Your Diabetes Treatment Changes

Almost immediately after giving birth, your body's insulin needs will decrease significantly. The extra hormones produced by the placenta that made your body resistant to the insulin you produced are now gone. No matter which type of diabetes you have, your regimen will change.

RETURNING TO PRE-PREGNANCY MEDICATIONS

Women with type 1 diabetes may find that they need little or no insulin for the first day or two after delivery, then more over the next few weeks but generally returning to something close to pre-pregnancy doses. As your body's requirements can change rapidly in the first few days after delivery, it is important to stay in close touch with your diabetes treatment team to monitor your therapy. Make sure you are checking your blood glucose levels often, as blood glucose levels tend to be erratic in the first few weeks after pregnancy. Within a few weeks, your insulin needs will stabilize and should be approximately the same as they were prior to pregnancy.

If you had type 2 diabetes before pregnancy and you were using insulin prior to pregnancy, you will probably need to continue using insulin. If you were using oral agents before pregnancy, whether you should return to your pre-pregnancy medication regimen for diabetes depends on whether or not that regimen was working well to keep your blood glucose levels in target.

Pregnancy, aging, and weight gain increase your insulin resistance. Now that your pregnancy is over, paying attention to achieving a healthy weight will help you manage your diabetes and help your medications or insulin work better.

Many women are surprised by how much their glucose control improved during pregnancy. Once you have succeeded in keeping your blood glucose levels in a target range, it is easier to believe in your ability to continue making healthy choices. Those healthy choices will serve you well for the rest of your life.

GESTATIONAL DIABETES

If you were diagnosed with gestational diabetes very early in pregnancy, you likely have type 2 diabetes and you may need to continue on medication. It's important to continue checking your blood glucose levels for a week or more after your baby is born to see if they stabilize. For most women with gestational diabetes found during the second trimester, delivery of your baby means blood glucose levels return to normal—for now. A woman who had gestational diabetes has a very high risk of developing type 2 diabetes—about a 50% chance in the next 10 years.

About four to six weeks after delivery, you should have testing to confirm that your gestational diabetes has gone away. The usual test to take is an oral glucose tolerance test. The oral glucose tolerance test will show whether your blood glucose levels are still in the diabetes range or have gone back to normal.

Occasionally the oral glucose tolerance test will show intermediate levels of glucose suggesting a condition called prediabetes. Prediabetes is a very strong risk factor for developing type 2 diabetes.

If you have prediabetes, you should know that weight loss (5–7% of your body weight) and exercise can delay or even prevent your condition from progressing to diabetes. If you have a history of gestational diabetes, whether or not you have prediabetes on your postpartum test, you should have an annual blood test to test for type 2 diabetes.

It is especially important for women with a new diagnosis of prediabetes or diabetes to make healthy choices and plan their next pregnancy well.

Follow-Up for Gestational Diabetes

If you had gestational diabetes your risk of developing type 2 diabetes over the 10 years following your pregnancy may be as high as 50%, even if your glucose test result within the 6 weeks following delivery is normal. You should continue to make healthy choices concerning meal planning, exercise, weight loss, and family planning. There is scientific evidence that if you can lose weight and maintain a regular exercise program you can prevent or delay the onset of type 2 diabetes. You will also need to have follow-up tests 4–6 weeks after delivery to make sure you don't still have diabetes. If your diabetes has gone away at that point, you need an annual blood test to check for type 2. These tests are crucial to helping you stay the healthiest mom you can be.

Losing Your Pregnancy Weight

Many women find that limiting their weight gain during pregnancy was difficult. Most women will find a 12–15 pound weight loss occurs without much effort in the first 2–3 weeks after delivery (due to losing the weight of the baby, placenta, and fluid retained toward the end of pregnancy). Beyond that, weight loss requires continuing effort.

Your long-term goal should be to achieve a healthy weight, not to just lose the weight that you gained during pregnancy. Knowing what a healthy weight is for your height may be determined from the table in chapter 5. A BMI over 30 is associated with increased long-term health risks including increased risk of developing type 2 diabetes, heart disease, high blood pressure, and other chronic medical problems, as well as future infertility and miscarriage. If you already have chronic medical complications and your BMI is over 35, you may even be a candidate to consider bariatric surgery (see chapter 2). Bariatric surgery can help you achieve a healthy weight, but it is not a quick fix. It requires significant changes in your lifestyle.

You should continue to follow your pregnancy meal plan or work with a dietitian to develop a new one. If you are breastfeeding, work with your dietitian to develop a meal plan that will balance your weight-loss plans with your breastfeeding nutrition needs.

Discuss your weight loss goals with your health care team after delivery. Pre-pregnancy weight, weight gain during pregnancy, desirable weight, breastfeeding status, age, and exercise levels should all be assessed to help figure out an appropriate weight-loss schedule, usually between 1–2 pounds per week. Gradual loss of weight is recommended and can be accomplished with a proper meal plan and exercise program. A more rapid weight loss is not recommended because it may contribute to fatigue and nutrient depletion.

Contraception and Family Planning

Now that you have your baby home, you should develop a family plan. You may want to have more children in the future, you may not plan on having more children, or you may not know what the future holds. No matter what your ideas are for the future, it's important to have a family plan. We talked in depth about family planning and contraception in chapter 2, but you will have some special needs specific to your body after delivery.

Your doctor will probably discourage you from resuming intercourse until your bleeding has stopped, your vaginal tissues (or, if you delivered by cesarean, your abdominal incision) have healed, and you have chosen a form of contraception. It is possible to ovulate and become pregnant much sooner after delivery than you would expect. Because it is possible to get pregnant before your 6 weeks' post-pregnancy visit to the doctor, it is a good idea to have a family planning method decided upon prior to leaving the hospital. Most family planning methods may be started in the days immediately following delivery, including the use of condoms, contraceptive foam, and the progesterone-only birth control pill. This last method is quite effective and will not decrease breast milk production or be harmful to your baby. It may, however, cause a slight increase in your blood glucose. Breastfeeding is not considered a reliable form of contraception after delivery.

If your family is complete and you don't want to have any more children, you may want to consider a permanent form of birth control, such as tubal sterilization. Do you have trouble taking medication on a daily basis? If so, a method such as the IUD that does not require your attention every day might be best for you. Are you worried about infections that could occur with a new partner? If so, then a barrier method might be best, either alone or in combination with another method. If none of these considerations apply to you, then you may choose a form of oral contraception such as the birth control pill. There are many forms of safe and effective contraception available today. Talk to your partner and your health care provider when making your decision, as there is no one "best method" for everybody. The "right" contraception for you is the one that is easy for you to use, is effective, and allows you to plan your future.

If you have type 1 or type 2 diabetes you will need to make sure your blood glucose is in a target range before getting pregnant again. If you had gestational diabetes or type 2 diabetes, you may need to lose weight or continue an exercise program to get yourself in the best possible health before trying to get pregnant.

Seeing your doctor to plan before your next pregnancy will significantly decrease your risk of experiencing complications related to diabetes in a future pregnancy. Remember that poor glucose control around and soon after the time of conception, before you may even realize you are pregnant, increases risks of birth defects and miscarriage. You can avoid this concern by working with your health care team to optimize your health and your medications prior to conception, and by not discontinuing your family planning method before your blood glucose levels and your overall health are in the best shape for carrying a pregnancy.

You may have found that managing gestational diabetes or diabetes during pregnancy took a lot of work. But there is a silver lining. You have learned how to take control of your health destiny and had the opportunity to develop healthy habits. Hopefully, you had a team of teachers—dietitians, doctors, and diabetes educators—to provide instruction and support. You have mastered the skills you need to continue your success. You may even find that your whole family has started to pay more attention to a healthy lifestyle. Now is the time to cement these positive changes in your family. If you can build upon this climate of achievement, you will be rewarded with better health. Use your new knowledge daily and keep up the good work!

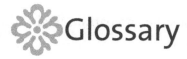# Glossary

A

A1C Test: A test that shows a person's average blood glucose levels over the past 2–3 months, usually shown as a percentage. The A1C measures the amount of hemoglobin to which glucose is attached (also called hemoglobin A1C) in the blood.

Abruption (abruptio placentae): Separation of the placenta from the uterus while the fetus is in the uterus. It can be life-threatening for the baby and requires emergency medical treatment.

ACE inhibitor: An oral medicine that lowers blood pressure. ACE stands for angiotensin-converting enzyme. For non-pregnant people with diabetes, especially those who have protein (albumin) in the urine, it also helps slow down kidney damage. Its use in pregnancy is not recommended, because of potential risks to the unborn baby.

American Diabetes Association (ADA): The nation's largest voluntary health organization dedicated to preventing and curing diabetes and improving the well-being of all people affected by diabetes.

Amniocentesis: A procedure to take fluid out of the amniotic sac for tests.

Amniotic fluid: The fluid filling the amniotic sac, in which the baby "floats."

Amniotic sac: Also known as the bag of waters. It is a fluid-filled sac that is attached to the placenta, in which the fetus develops.

Angiotensin receptor blocker (ARB): An oral medication that is used to treat hypertension. As with the ACE inhibitors, it is recommended to not use these medications during pregnancy.

Antepartum: Before delivery. An example would be antepartum fetal monitoring or testing the fetus before delivery.

B

Basal insulin: An intermediate- or long-acting insulin that is absorbed slowly and gives the body a steady, low level of insulin to manage blood glucose levels between meals, thus mimicking the body's natural low-level steady background release of insulin.

Bilirubin: A waste product of red blood cells that is excreted by the liver. Elevated bilirubin in the blood causes jaundice.

Biophysical profile: A test of fetal health that combines a sonogram with a non-stress test. The biophysical profile evaluates fetal movement, muscle tone, and breathing as well as the amount of amniotic fluid present.

Blood glucose: The main sugar found in the body and the body's main energy source; also called blood sugar.

Blood glucose level: the amount of glucose in a given amount of blood; often measured in milligrams of glucose per deciliter of blood and written as mg/dl.

Blood glucose meter: A small, portable machine used by people with diabetes to frequently check their blood glucose levels. After pricking the skin with a lancet, one places a drop of blood on a test strip in the machine, and then the meter displays the blood glucose level on a digital display.

Blood pressure: The force of blood exerted on the inside walls of blood vessels. It is expressed as a ratio (e.g., 120/80 mmHg, read as 120 over 80 in millimeters of mercury). The first number is the systolic pressure—or pressure when the heart pushes blood out of the arteries—and the second number is the diastolic pressure—the pressure when the heart rests.

Body mass index (BMI): A method of evaluating the body's weight relative to its height and represented as weight in kilograms divided by the square of the height in meters. (kg/m^2); used to determine the following categories: underweight, normal, overweight, and obese.

Bolus insulin: An extra amount of insulin taken to cover an expected rise in blood glucose, often related to a meal or snack.

C

Carbohydrate: One of the three primary nutrients found in food; primarily starches, vegetables, fruits, dairy products, and sugars.

Cervix: The opening of the uterus into the vagina.

Cesarean delivery (also called cesarean section or cesarean birth): An operation where an incision is made through the abdomen and uterus, through which the baby is removed. Cesarean delivery is usually performed if the baby cannot be delivered by the usual vaginal route.

Continuous glucose monitor (CGM): A device that continuously records blood glucose levels throughout the day and night through a subcutaneously implanted sensor. The sensor must be replaced about every three days. The system is used to measure blood glucose levels in order to help identify fluctuations and trends that would otherwise go unnoticed with standard A1C tests and fingerstick measurements.

Contraction stress test (CST): Also called an oxytocin challenge test (OCT). This is a test where the mother's uterus is stimulated to have a few mild contractions while the doctor monitors the fetus's heartbeat. The small amount of contraction is not enough to cause labor and usually stops as soon as the oxytocin is discontinued.

D

Diabetes mellitus: A group of diseases with one common factor: elevated blood glucose (sugar). Diabetes may be caused by one or a combination of several changes in the body, including decreased secretion of insulin by the pancreas, high levels of hormones that act against insulin, or resistance of the body to insulin.

Diabetologist: A physician, usually an internist or endocrinologist, who specializes in the treatment of diabetes mellitus.

Dietetic: A term often used in advertising that means one ingredient has been changed. It may mean fewer calories, less fat, less sugar, or less salt. It does not mean the same as diabetic, which usually refers to products containing less sugar or a different kind of sugar.

Dietitian: A health professional with special training in nutrition. A Registered Dietitian (R.D.) has met the high standards of The American Dietetic Association.

E

Endocrinologist: An internist specializing in endocrine and metabolic diseases, including diabetes mellitus.

Exercise: Any form of movement that burns energy.

F

Fat: One of the main nutrients in food. Fats are the body's major storage system for energy. Dietary fats include margarine, shortening, oils, and butter.

Fetal monitor: A machine that records contractions of the mother's uterus and her baby's heartbeat. The machine is capable of recording from devices strapped on to the mother's abdomen or placed through her vagina and attached to the baby's scalp. The second method cannot be used until the bag of waters has broken.

Fetal surveillance or fetal monitoring: A term describing tests of fetal well-being performed at varying times during the pregnancy. These tests include the biophysical profile, contraction stress test, and non-stress test.

Fetus: Term used for the developing baby while it is still in the mother's uterus.

Fiber: Fiber is the indigestible portion of plant foods, such as the outer layer of grains or the woody part of many vegetables.

G

Gastric bypass: A bariatric surgical procedure in which the stomach is made smaller and digestion bypasses part of the small intestine; often done to help patients lose a large amount of body weight.

Gestation: Pregnancy.

Gestational age: Age of the baby from the beginning of pregnancy. For example, after seven months of pregnancy, the baby's gestational age is 28 weeks.

Gestational diabetes: A type of diabetes that develops only during pregnancy and usually disappears upon delivery, but increases the risk that the mother will later develop diabetes; managed with meal planning, physical activity, and sometimes insulin.

Glucagon: A hormone produced by the alpha cells in the pancreas that raises blood glucose levels. An injectable form of glucagon, available by prescription, may be used to treat severe hypoglycemia.

Glucose: One of the simplest forms of sugar; a simple sugar found in blood that serves as the body's main source of energy.

Glucose challenge test: A screening test for gestational diabetes usually done between the 24th and 28th week of pregnancy.

Glucose tolerance test: The definitive test to diagnose gestational diabetes. Blood glucose tests are taken each hour for two or three hours after drinking a liquid containing a fixed amount of glucose.

H

Hormone: A chemical made by one cell or organ (gland) that is carried (usually in the bloodstream) to another cell or organ where it works.

Hyperglycemia: High blood glucose. Symptoms include excessive thirst, excessive urination, and excessive hunger.

Hypoglycemia: Low blood glucose. Symptoms include nervousness, hunger, dizziness, shakiness, perspiration, lightheadedness, and confusion.

Hypoglycemia unawareness: A state in which a person does not feel or recognize the symptoms of low blood glucose.

I

Injection site rotation: The process of changing among several different places on the body where an injection is administered; prevents the formation of scar tissue.

Insulin: A hormone secreted by cells in the pancreas. Insulin lowers the level of sugar in the blood. Insulin is also a medicine that is used to treat diabetes.

Insulin pen: A device for injecting insulin. It resembles a fountain pen and holds replaceable cartridges of insulin. A dial is often used to set the insulin dose. Some pens are disposable.

Insulin pump: An insulin-delivering device about the size of a deck of cards that can be worn on a belt or kept in a pocket. It carries a reservoir of insulin connected to narrow, flexible tubing that ends with a needle that is inserted just under the skin. Users set the pump to give a basal amount of insulin continuously throughout the day. Based on programming done by the user, pumps also release bolus insulin to cover meals and at other times when blood glucose levels are high.

Insulin resistance: A condition characterized by the body's inability to respond to and use the insulin that it produces, meaning that insulin cannot function properly and higher levels of insulin are needed to achieve the same effects. This can result in high blood glucose levels and high levels of insulin in the blood.

Intermediate-acting insulin: A type of insulin that starts to lower blood glucose levels within 1–2 hours after injection and has its strongest effects 6–12 hours after injection, depending on the type used.

Intravenous: Fluids and/or medications given directly into the bloodstream through a vein.

J

Jaundice (hyperbilirubinemia): Yellowing of the skin and eyes caused by increased levels of bilirubin.

K

Ketone: An acid product of fat breakdown. It is produced if there is not enough carbohydrate in the diet. It is also produced if insulin levels are too low.

L

Labor: Muscular contractions in the uterus that squeeze down to deliver the baby.

Long-acting insulin: A basal insulin that starts to lower blood glucose levels within 4–6 hours after injection and has its strongest effects 10–18 hours after injection.

M

Macrosomia: Describes a baby who is abnormally large.

Malformation: Birth defect.

N

Neonate: Newborn baby.

Neonatologist: A pediatrician who specializes in the care of the newborn.

Nonstress test (NST): A test of fetal well-being. The NST is done by monitoring fetal heartbeat changes while the mother lies quietly on an examination table.

NPH: An intermediate-acting insulin.

Nurse educator: A nurse who has additional training and special interest in diabetes education.

O

Obstetrician: A physician specializing in the care of pregnant women and delivering babies.

Oxytocin: A hormone from the pituitary gland, which stimulates the uterus to contract. It is also a medication used in small doses to stimulate mild contractions in the contraction stress test. Larger amounts are used to induce or stimulate labor.

P

Pancreas: An organ located in the abdomen behind the stomach and small intestine. The pancreas makes enzymes for digestion in the intestines and also secretes many hormones, including insulin, into the bloodstream.

Pediatrician: A physician who specializes in the care of infants and children.

Perinatal: Around the time of delivery.

Perinatologist: An obstetrician specializing in the care of complicated pregnancies. Also called a high-risk pregnancy specialist and a specialist in maternal-fetal medicine.

Placenta: A specialized organ directly connected to both the mother's and fetus's blood vessels. The placenta gets nutrients from the mother's blood for the fetus and secretes hormones necessary for normal pregnancy.

Polycystic ovary syndrome (PCOS): A hormonal disorder that affects women of reproductive age and which can cause infertility in some patients. Many patients with this disorder also have insulin resistance. Some symptoms include infrequent or absent periods, acne, obesity, and excess hair growth.

Postpartum: After delivery.

Preeclampsia: A serious disease in which pregnant women develop hypertension, and develop protein in the urine. It is more common in women with diabetes.

Prematurity: Birth of a baby before the full term of pregnancy is complete—usually used to describe any birth before 39 weeks of pregnancy.

Protein: One of the main nutrients in food. Protein are the building blocks of muscle, bone, etc. Proteins are made up of amino acids.

Examples of foods high in protein are: meat, poultry, fish, cheese, milk, eggs, and dried beans.

R

Rapid-acting insulin: A type of insulin that starts to lower blood glucose levels within 5–10 minutes after injection and has its strongest effects 30 minutes to 3 hours after injection, depending on the type used.

Respiratory distress syndrome (RDS): A disease of the lungs causing breathing difficulty in the newborn baby. RDS is more common in premature babies and in the children of mothers with poorly controlled diabetes.

S

Short-acting insulin: A type of insulin that starts to lower blood glucose within 30 minutes after injection and has its strongest effect 2–5 hours after injection.

Starvation ketosis: A form of ketosis occurring when not enough carbohydrates are eaten.

Sterilization: An operation to make a man or woman permanently unable to have children. This is usually done by an operation called a vasectomy (for men) or a tubal ligation (for women).

T

Trimester: One-third of the pregnancy. The first trimester includes weeks 1–12; the second, weeks 13–26; and the third, weeks 27–40.

Tubal ligation: An operation to cut the Fallopian tubes that carry the egg from the ovary to the uterus. As in a vasectomy, tubal ligation does not affect sexual function. (Also called tubal sterilization.)

Type 1 diabetes: This occurs when the pancreas can no longer secrete insulin. It is more common in young people, but can occur at any age. Type 1 diabetes must be treated with insulin.

Type 2 diabetes: A type of high blood sugar that occurs when the pancreas may still secrete insulin but the body is resistant to normal insulin levels. Type 2 diabetes may be treated with diet alone, diet and exercise, or diet, exercise, and oral drugs or insulin.

U

Ultrasound (sonogram): A sound wave picture of the fetus, placenta, and uterus. Ultrasound makes a picture of the area studied by bouncing sound waves off the organ being visualized.

Uterus: Womb.

V

Vaginal delivery: Delivery of the baby through the vagina.

Vasectomy: An operation to cut the tubes that carry sperm from the testicles to the penis. Vasectomy does not affect sex drive or the ability to have intercourse.

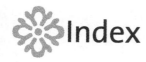Index

condoms, 22, 110
constipation, 75–76
continuous glucose monitors
(CGMs), 48–49
contraception, 20–23, 109–111
contraction stress test (CST), 39

D

delivery (of baby), 87–92
Depo-Provera, 21
detemir (Levemir), 59, 60
DHA, 77–78
diabetes care providers, 35
Diabetes Forecast, 48
diabetes generally
  complications of, 9, 13
  defined, 8
  diagnosis of, 13–14
  effects on pregnancy, 7–9,
    15–16, 39–42, 49
  statistics, 8
  types of, 9–13
diabetic ketoacidosis, 50–51
diaphragms, 22
dietitians, 35
Down syndrome screening, 37

E

emergency contraception, 23
exercise
  activities to avoid, 82
  benefits of, 11, 30, 71, 81, 106
  post-bariatric surgery, 28
  pregnancy-specific, 46–47,
    81–82

F

family planning, 21, 109–111
fasting glucose level test, 14
fetal echocardiogram, 38
fetal monitoring, 38, 90–91
fetal well-being tests, 38–39
fish oil, 77–78
folic acid, 29
food cravings, 74

G

garlic, 78
gastric bypass surgery, 28–29
gestational diabetes
  breast feeding and, 97–99
  described, 12–13
  follow-up for, 108
  insulin needs of, 47, 57, 65,
    107–108 (*See also* insulin)
  meal planning, 77
  post-delivery, 96–97
  pregnancy-related
    complications, 15–16, 49
  weight management and, 79–80
ginger, 78
ginkgo, 78
ginseng, 78
glargine (Lantus), 59, 60
glucagon, 53
glucose tablets, 52
glulisine (Apidra), 59
glyburide, 66–67

L

labor, delivery, 87–92
Lantus (glargine), 59, 60
Levemir (detemir), 59, 60
lispro (Humalog), 59

M

magnesium deficiency, 100
medications, 66–67, 92, 97–98,
      107–108
metformin, 66–67
morning sickness, 75

N

nausea, 75
nephropathy, 38, 41
neuropathy, 40
non stress test (NST), 39
Novolin, 59
Novolog (aspart), 59
NPH insulin, 59, 60, 76
nutrition
      benefits of, 71, 106
      beverages, 74
      blood glucose management
          (*See* blood glucose
          management)
      carbohydrates, 46, 52, 73, 76–77
      constipation, 75–76
      food cravings, 74
      heartburn, 76
      insulin and, 76–77 (*See also*
          insulin)
      morning sickness, 75
      overview, 71–73

plate method, 73
post-bariatric surgery, 28
protein requirements, 72
supplements, 29–30, 77–78

O

obstetricians, 35
omega-3 fatty acids, 77–78
oral (hormonal) contraception, 21,
      109–111
oral glucose tolerance test, 14, 108
oral medications, 66–67, 92, 97–98,
      107–108

P

phototherapy, 100
placental function testing, 38
planning, preparation
      birth control methods, 20–23,
          109–111
      exercise (*See* exercise)
      health goals, 30
      nutrition (*See* nutrition)
      overview, 19–20, 110
      pre-pregnancy exam, 24–25
      unexpected pregnancy, 23–24
      weight management, 26–29, 47,
          78–80, 109
plasma glucose level test, 14
plate method, 73
polycythemia, 100
post-delivery care, 95–101
postpartum depression, 106
prediabetes, 108
preeclampsia, 16, 41, 42, 49, 89
pregnancy

diabetes effects on, 7–9, 15–16,
    39–42, 49
effects on insulin resistance,
    12–13, 57, 58, 71–72, 107
fetal well-being tests, 38—39
pre-pregnancy exam, 23–25
stages, 33–34
unexpected, preparation for,
    23–24

R

ReliOn, 59
respiratory distress syndrome
    (RDS), 100–101
retinopathy, 38, 40
rule of 15, 52–53

S

sexual intercourse, 110
shoulder dystocia, 89
special care, 33–39
spina bifida, 38
sponges, 22
spontaneous labor, 88
sterilization, 23, 110

T

Tachypnea of the Newborn
    (TTN), 101
testing
    A1C, 14, 24–25
    contraction stress test (CST),
        39
    fasting glucose level, 14
    fetal well-being, 38—39
    kick count, 38–39

non stress test (NST), 39
oral glucose tolerance, 14, 108
placental function, 38
plasma glucose level, 14
thyroid, 42
type 1 diabetes
    described, 10–12
    insulin needs of, 47, 57–58, 65,
        107 (*See also* insulin)
    placental function testing, 38
    pregnancy planning (*See*
        planning, preparation)
    pregnancy-related
        complications, 15, 49
    pre-pregnancy exam, 24–25
type 2 diabetes
    described, 9–10
    insulin needs of, 47, 57–58,
        65–66, 107 (*See also*
        insulin)
    medications post-delivery, 96
    pregnancy planning (*See*
        planning, preparation)
    pregnancy-related
        complications, 15, 49
    risk factors, 13, 97

U

ultrasounds, 36–38

W

weight management, 26–29, 47,
    78–80, 109

Other Titles from the American Diabetes Association

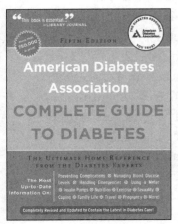

Complete Guide to Diabetes, 5th Edition

by American Diabetes Association
Have all the tips and information on diabetes that you need close at hand. The world's largest collection of diabetes self-care tips, techniques, and tricks for solving diabetes-related problems is back in its fifth edition, and it's bigger and better than ever before.
Order no. 4809-05; Price $22.95

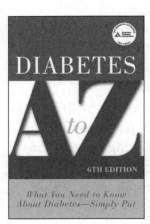

Diabetes A to Z, 6th Edition

by American Diabetes Association
If you want the ins and outs of diabetes without the confusing jargon, then *Diabetes A to Z* is your go-to resource. *Diabetes A to Z*, 6th Edition, contains the most up-to-date recommendations by the American Diabetes Association, presented in a simple, yet informative, format. Get your answers to all your questions quickly and get back to living your life.
Order no. 4801-06; Price $16.95

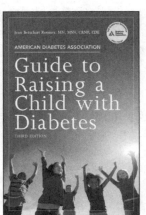

Guide to Raising a Child with Diabetes

Jean Betschart Roemer, MN, MSN, CRNP, CDE
Guide to Raising a Child with Diabetes, 3rd Edition, is an invaluable parenting tool, featuring the latest advances in diabetes care, plus parenting advice from diabetes experts. Learn to navigate through the normal activities of childhood and raise your kids to be strong, confident, and capable of managing their own diabetes care.
Order no. 4901-03; Price $18.95

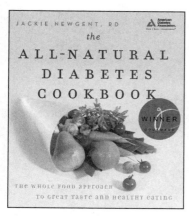

The All-Natural Diabetes Cookbook

by Jackie Newgent, RD

Instead of relying on artificial sweeteners or not-so-real substitutions to reduce calories, sugar, and fat, *The All-Natural Diabetes Cookbook* takes a different approach, focusing on naturally delicious fresh foods and whole-food ingredients to create fantastic meals that deliver amazing taste and well-rounded nutrition. And absolutely nothing is artificial.

Order no. 4663-01; Price $18.95

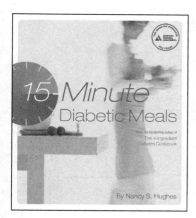

15-Minute Diabetic Meals

by Nancy S. Hughes

What can you cook in 15 minutes? It's time to find out! With over 200 time-saving recipes, *15-Minute Diabetic Meals* shows you how to cut corners by using convenience items and making smart choices at the grocery store to make healthy meals in a snap. You'll be amazed at what you can prepare in absolutely no time.

Order no. 4676-01; Price $18.95

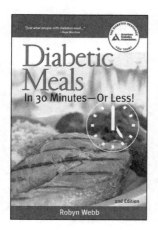

Diabetic Meals in 30 Minutes—or Less!

by Robyn Webb

For over 10 years, *Diabetic Meals in 30 Minutes—Or Less!* has helped people with diabetes eat well. Now, in this revised second edition, learn how to create, plan, and serve healthy, quick meals every day of every week. Healthy eating for the person with diabetes doesn't have to take up every minute—save that extra time to enjoy your tasty food!

Order no. 4614-02; Price $14.95

To order these and other great American Diabetes Association titles, call **1-800-232-6733** or visit **http://shopdiabetes.org**. American Diabetes Association titles are also available in bookstores nationwide.